Pharmacology
for the **Surgical**
Technologist

Pharmacology
for the Surgical
Technologist

Katherine Snyder, CST, BS

Program Director and Instructor
Surgical Technology
Presentation College
Aberdeen, South Dakota

Chris Keegan, CST, MS

Assistant Professor and Chairman
Department of Surgical Technology
Vincennes University
Vincennes, Indiana

W.B. Saunders Company

A Division of Harcourt Brace & Company

Philadelphia London Toronto Montreal Sydney Tokyo

W. B. SAUNDERS COMPANY
A Division of Harcourt Brace & Company

The Curtis Center
Independence Square West
Philadelphia, Pennsylvania 19106

NOTICE

Surgical Technology is an ever-changing field. Standard safety precautions must be followed, but as new research and clinical experience broaden our knowledge, changes in treatment and drug therapy become necessary or appropriate. Readers are advised to check the product information currently provided by the manufacturer of each drug to be administered to verify the recommended dose, the method and duration of administration, and the contraindications. It is the responsibility of the treating physician, relying on experience and knowledge of the patient, to determine dosages and the best treatment for the patient. Neither the publisher nor the editor assumes any responsibility for any injury and/or damage to persons or property.

The Publisher

LIMITS OF LEGAL AUTHORITY

The limits of legal authority for the surgical technologist to act or perform the indicated roles described in this textbook are controlled by each individual state through its statutes, case law, regulatory law, attorney general opinions, and medical licensing boards. Discussion of these sources of law for each state is beyond the scope of this text. Except as otherwise noted, this book describes the general practice of surgical technology in the United States, not the legal authority for such practice. It is the surgical technologist's responsibility to consult the limitations on his/her role in acts described in this book for his/her area.

Library of Congress Cataloging-in-Publication Data

Snyder, Katherine.
    Pharmacology for the surgical technologist / Katherine Snyder,
Chris Keegan. — 1st ed.
       p.   cm.
    ISBN 0–7216–6321–4
    1. Pharmacology. 2. Operating room technicians. I. Keegan,
Chris. II. Title.
    [DNLM: 1. Pharmaceutical Preparations—administration & dosage
nurses' instruction. 2. Pharmacology—methods nurses' instruction.
3. Perioperative Nursing—methods. 4. Operating Room Technicians.
QV 748 S675p 1999]
RM300.S638 1999
615'.1—dc21
DNLM/DLC   98–33323

PHARMACOLOGY FOR THE SURGICAL TECHNOLOGIST   ISBN 0–7216–6321–4

Printed in the United States of America.

Last digit is the print number: 9 8 7 6 5 4 3 2

This book is dedicated to the memory of Dorothy M. Kadlec, CST, teacher, mentor, and friend who, by example, taught me to practice the profession of surgical technology with dignity and integrity.

Kathy Snyder

This book is dedicated to Dr. Stephen C. Ferguson, "Fergie," my boss, teacher, mentor, and friend who encouraged me and helped me to grow in my career and profession.

Chris Keegan

Preface

A few years ago, a committee of instructors met to work on revisions to the *Core Curriculum for Surgical Technology*. During the meeting, the topic of textbooks surfaced—in particular pharmacology textbooks. It generally was agreed that no adequate pharmacology textbook for surgical technologists existed. As the discussion progressed and we complained about the situation, a question was posed: "Well, are you going to be part of the problem or part of the solution?" This textbook is our response to that question. It offers, for the first time in a single text, a distinct combination of subject matter. The text is organized into three units, each focusing on information specific to the surgical environment. Students will review basic math skills and learn a framework of pharmacologic principles in order to apply the information in surgical situations; learn commonly used medications by category, with frequent descriptions of actual surgical applications; and learn basic anesthesia concepts, not previously presented at this level, in order to function more effectively as a surgical team member.

Special learning tools used in this text include:

- Definitions of Key Terms, which are then boldfaced in the chapters
- Learning Objectives, stated at the beginning of each chapter
- Insight boxes that offer additional information on the subject matter
- Illustrations, including real surgical photographs, designed to familiarize the student with the surgical environment
- Tables that condense information, to facilitate learning
- Chapter summaries that emphasize critical content
- Review questions at the end of each chapter that provide opportunities for critical thinking

These features have been developed to assist the student in learning this new and often unfamiliar material. Key terms are defined at the beginning of each chapter for quick reference, and students are encouraged to use a medical dictionary as needed for routine medical terminology used throughout the text. Learning objectives are used to guide the students through the material, emphasizing important concepts. Chapter review questions are designed to help students think about concepts from a broader perspective, or to apply content at a more personal level, particularly their local clinical facility.

The authors would appreciate comments and suggestions from practitioners, instructors, and students using this text. Please contact us through W.B. Saunders Company, The Curtis Center, Independence Square West, Philadelphia, PA 19106–3399.

Acknowledgments

We would like to acknowledge and sincerely thank the following people for their valuable input and assistance in the development and completion of this project. Thanks to the staff at W.B. Saunders for sharing our vision and for helping us make that vision a reality. We are especially grateful to Selma Kaszczuk and Rachael Kelly for their patience and guidance throughout the entire project. Thanks to our students for good-naturedly using various drafts of this text and for their helpful input. Our special thanks to Dorothy Corrigan, CST, for asking "the question" and to the staff and members of the Association of Surgical Technologists for their encouragement and assistance.

Kathy wishes to thank the following people for their varied roles in the development of this book. First, my parents, Gus and Eileen, for giving me the gift of life. My sons, Bryan and Eric, for their patience and cooperation. Curt Pudwill, CRNA, for pointing me in the right direction. Gretchen Wienecke, MD, and Simon Body, MD, for reviewing early drafts of the anesthesia chapters and providing excellent suggestions. Brook, Jenny, Melissa, and Shannon for using the earliest draft and making such helpful comments. Kevin, Sandy, Melissa, Trena, Frank, Mary, and St. Luke's–Midland Regional Medical Center for help with photographs. And above all, thanks to Almighty God; Father, Son, and Holy Spirit, the generous source of all the gifts in my life. I offer this work in thanksgiving for those blessings and I pray that this work will ultimately benefit the surgical patient through the competent care of professional surgical technologists. To God be all the glory and honor.

Chris would sincerely like to thank the following people for their generous contributions, advice, guidance, and review of chapters. Without their expertise, this text would not have been possible. Physicians who took time from their busy schedules to answer questions are: Donald Cobb, MD, Edward Daetwyler, MD, Duane Kuhlenschmidt, MD, Joseph Meyer, MD, Timothy Williams, DO, William Penland, MD, and Frederick Sigda, MD. Educators who gave insights and reviews are: Daniel Scavone, PhD, Professor of History, University of Southern Indiana; Larry Barchett, MA, Professor, Math and Science Division, Vincennes University; Sandra Stewart, MS, Professor, Math and Science Division, Vincennes University; and Elizabeth Slagle, RN, MS, Chair and

Instructor, Surgical Technology Program, University of St. Francis. The staff from the Learning Resource Center at Vincennes University who helped with research and guidance are: Joseph Helms, Richard King, Robert Slayton, and David Fischer. Hospitals that generously donated supplies, equipment, and facilities are: Good Samaritan Hospital, Vincennes, Indiana; and St. Mary's Medical Center, Evansville, Indiana. And last, but not least, Vincennes University and Marjorie Miller, MS Hed, MSN, Dean, Health Occupations Division, for constant support and encouragement during this project. On a more personal level, my love and gratitude to my husband Jack and daughter Kim. Through them, dreams come true.

Contents

UNIT **ONE**

Introduction to Pharmacology

As a surgical technologist, you'll mix and measure medications and deliver them to and from the sterile field. This means you'll be dealing with *pharmacology*—the science of drugs. In Unit I, then, we'll look at general pharmacologic information, including how drugs are measured, what kinds of drugs there are, what laws pertain to them, and how they're administered. In Chapter 1, we focus on precision because it's critical to deliver exactly the right quantity and strength of any drug. Thus, we review the mathematics you'll need to do that job. We include a quick refresher on basic computational techniques and a review of the measurement systems used in medicine. It's also critical to be accurate—you have to deliver the right drug in the right form. So Chapter 2 gives you a look at the drugs themselves—their sources, names, and classifications as well as the routes by which they're administered and the forms they come in. This chapter, then, provides a framework of pharmacologic terms, concepts, and principles—a framework that helps you understand current information about drugs and prepares you to assimilate new information effectively. In Chapter 3, we focus on laws and regulations. You'll see why we have drug laws, what kinds of laws there are, and what government agencies enforce them. Then, in Chapter 4, we concentrate on the methods you'll use when handling drugs, including aseptic practice, proper drug identification, and clear labeling.

CHAPTER **1**

Basic Mathematics

OBJECTIVES

Upon completion of this chapter, you should be able to:

1 Define terminology, abbreviations, and symbols used in basic mathematics and measurement systems.
2 Read and write Roman numerals accurately.
3 Convert between Arabic and Roman numerals.
4 Use fractions in conversions and calculations.
5 Read and write decimals.
6 Use decimals in conversions and calculations.
7 Convert between fractions and decimals.

8 Explain the meaning of percentages.

9 Convert between percentages and decimals, and between percentages and fractions.

10 Explain ratios and proportions.

11 Use ratios and proportions to solve problems.

12 Convert temperatures between the Fahrenheit and Celsius scales.

13 Recognize different measurement systems and explain their uses.

14 Identify equivalent values between measurement systems.

KEY TERMS

Apothecary system An archaic system for measuring fluids and solids based on the minim (a unit of volume) and the grain (a unit of weight).

Arabic numerals A system of writing numbers based on ten integers: 1, 2, 3, 4, 5, 6, 7, 8, 9, and 0. Used for counting, measuring, and calculation.

Celsius scale A temperature scale in which the difference between the freezing point and boiling point of water is divided into 100 degrees, so that water freezes at 0°C and boils at 100°C. Also known as the centigrade scale.

Decimal point A place holder that separates numbers greater than 1 from numbers less than 1 in the decimal system.

Fahrenheit scale A temperature scale in which the difference between the freezing point and boiling point of water is divided into 180 degrees, so that water freezes at 32°F and boils at 212°F.

Metric system A decimal system of weights and measures based on the meter, liter, and gram, universally used for scientific measurements.

Proportion A statement of equality between two ratios; an equation whose members are ratios.

Ratio The relation between two quantities expressed as a quotient; the relative sizes of two numbers or quantities.

Roman numerals A system of writing numbers based on the ancient Roman counting system using seven basic letter characters—I, V, X, L, C, D, and M— to express the tally quantities 1, 5, 10, 50, 100, 500, and 1000, respectively.

In this chapter we look at basic mathematics, including Roman numerals, fractions, decimals, percents, and ratios and proportions. We'll review how to solve simple problems, perform fundamental calculations, and make important conversions. Many surgical technology students are already familiar with these principles, this chapter is designed as a "brush-up" for students who need to refresh their mathematical skills. Each rule is explained, then examples are given to illustrate its principle. In addition, simple exercises allow students to practice the rules they have just reviewed. Specific surgical technology story problems are placed throughout the chapter to give students an opportunity to test knowledge in realistic situations. In addition to math, this chapter introduces the student to three systems of measurement. Students use basic mathematical skills to perform conversions between systems of measurement. Knowledge of metric measurements and basic mathematical skills necessary in pharmacology are also used during surgical procedures, particularly when using implants and various grafts.

Roman Numerals

Unlike the familiar **Arabic numerals** (0, 1, 2, 3, 4, 5, 6, 7, 8, 9), which are commonly used in mathematical calculations and measurements, **Roman numerals** are used only for counting. Seven basic symbols—I, V, X, L, C, D, M—stand for the whole numbers 1, 5, 10, 50, 100, 500, and 1000; and combinations of these symbols are used to indicate quantities in prescriptions. (See Table 1–1.)

Reading Roman Numerals

To read Roman numerals, look at the order of the characters; then add or subtract.
- When a Roman numeral character *precedes* another of greater value, its value is *subtracted* from the greater one.
- When a Roman numeral character *follows* another of greater value, its value is *added* to the greater one.

Examples

(1) IX = (10 − 1) = 9
(2) XI = (10 + 1) = 11
(3) XIV = [10 + (5 − 1)] =14

TABLE 1–1 Roman Numerals

Roman numerals	Arabic numerals	Roman numerals	Arabic numerals	Roman numerals	Arabic numerals
ss, s̄s̄	1/2	**X**	10	**C**	100
I	1	XV	15	**D**	500
II	2	XX	20	**M**	1000
III	3	XXX	30		
IV	4	XL	40		
V	5	**L**	50		
VI	6	LX	60		
VII	7	LXX	70		
VIII	8	LXXX	80		
IX	9	XC	90		

④ XVI = [10 + (5 + 1)] = 16
⑤ DLV = [500 + (50 + 5)] = 555

- When Roman numeral characters of *equal value* are in sequence, their values are *added.* (Numerals are never repeated in a sequence more than three times.)

Examples

① III = (1 + 1 + 1) = 3
② XXX = (10 + 10 + 10) = 30
③ CCC = (100 + 100 + 100) = 300
④ CII = [100 + (1 + 1)] = 102

☞ Use two letters to represent a Roman numeral rather than three when possible. For example, XV denotes 15 (not VVV) and CL denotes 150 (not LLL).

- When a Roman numeral is placed between two others of greater value, its value is subtracted from the numeral following it.

Examples

① XIX = [10 + (10 − 1)] = 19
② LXXXIX = [50 + 10 + 10 + 10 + (10 − 1)] = 89
③ CLXIV = [100 + 50 + 10 + (5 − 1)] = 164
④ CXC = [100 + (100 − 10)] = 190
⑤ DXLIX = [500 + (50 − 10) + (10 − 1)] = 549

EXERCISES

1. Convert the following Arabic numerals to Roman numerals:

a. $\frac{1}{2}$ = _____   f. 102 = _____

b. 10 = _____   g. 1005 = _____

c. 7 = _____   h. 608 = _____

d. 40 = _____   i. 975 = _____

e. 66 = _____   j. 404 = _____

2. Convert the following Roman numerals to Arabic numerals:

a. LXV = _____   f. MCMXCIV = _____

b. MCM = _____   g. CCXC = _____

c. XVIII = _____   h. DCLIX = _____

d. DCC = _____   i. MI = _____

e. LD = _____   j. MMMDCCLIII = _____

Fractions

A *fraction* is a quotient—a number that can be written in an *a/b* or $\frac{a}{b}$ form, where *b* is never equal to 0. We say that *a* and *b* are the *terms* of the fraction where *a* is the *numerator* and *b* is the *denominator*.

Example

One-half = 1/2 = $\frac{1}{2}$ =

$\dfrac{1}{2}$ $a = 1$ is the numerator
      $b = 2$ is the denominator

Five-sixths = 5/6 = $\frac{5}{6}$ =

$\dfrac{5}{6}$ $a = 5$ is the numerator
      $b = 6$ is the denominator

Five-eighths = 5/8 = $\frac{5}{8}$ =

$\dfrac{5}{8}$ $a = 5$ is the numerator
      $b = 8$ is the denominator

We use fractions to express division of a whole into equal parts:

- The denominator tells how many equal parts into which the whole is divided.
- The numerator tells how many of those equal parts we're interested in.

Example

Imagine a pie divided into 6 equal parts, and 5 of those equal parts are eaten.

$\dfrac{5}{6}$ number of eaten parts
      number of equal parts into which the whole pie is divided

So

- $\frac{5}{6}$ of the pie is eaten
- $\frac{1}{6}$ of the pie remains

The larger the denominator, the smaller the pieces (fractions) in the whole.

☞ $\frac{1}{2}$ is greater than $\frac{1}{3}$

$\frac{1}{3}$ is greater than $\frac{1}{4}$

$\frac{1}{4}$ is greater than $\frac{1}{5}$

$\frac{1}{3}$ is greater than $\frac{1}{6}$

and so on

Example

Imagine a circle divided into 8 equal parts, and 5 of those equal parts are shaded.

$\frac{5}{8}$ number of shaded equal parts

    number of equal parts into which the whole circle is divided

So

- $\frac{5}{8}$ of the circle is shaded
- $\frac{3}{8}$ of the circle is not shaded

If the numerator and denominator are equal to each other, the fraction is equal to 1.

Example

$\frac{1}{1} = \quad \frac{2}{2} = \quad \frac{5}{5} = \quad \frac{100}{100} = \quad \frac{3569}{3569} = 1$

If the numerator is less than the denominator, the value of the fraction is less than 1. Then the fraction is a *proper fraction*.

Example

$\frac{2}{3} \quad \frac{3}{4} \quad \frac{3}{5} \quad \frac{99}{100}$

If the numerator is greater than the denominator, the value of the fraction is more than 1. Then the fraction is an *improper fraction*.

Example

$$\frac{3}{2} \qquad \frac{4}{3} \qquad \frac{12}{6} \qquad \frac{15}{10}$$

A *mixed number* is a combination of a whole number with a fraction.

Example

$$1\frac{1}{2} \qquad 2\frac{1}{3} \qquad 5\frac{3}{7} \qquad 8\frac{49}{50}$$

You can change a mixed number to an improper fraction in three steps. Given a mixed number $2\frac{1}{2}$,

> **Step 1:** Multiply the denominator of the fraction by the whole number:
>
> $$\text{Whole number} \times \text{denominator} = 2 \times 2 = 4$$
>
> **Step 2:** Add the numerator to the result obtained in Step 1:
>
> $$\text{Numerator} + (\text{Step 1 result}) = 1 + 4 = 5$$
>
> **Step 3:** Use the result obtained in Step 2 as the numerator of the new fraction; use the original denominator as the new denominator:
>
> $$\frac{\text{Step 2 result}}{\text{Original denominator}} = \frac{5}{2} = \frac{5}{2}$$

Thus, the mixed number $2\frac{1}{2}$ is the same as the improper fraction $\frac{5}{2}$.
You can change an improper fraction to a mixed number in 4 steps.
Given an improper fraction $\frac{8}{5}$,

> **Step 1:** Divide the numerator by the denominator:
>
> $$\frac{\text{Numerator}}{\text{Denominator}} = \frac{8}{5} = 1\text{ R3} \qquad (\text{i.e., 1 with 3 left over})$$
>
> **Step 2:** Use the whole number obtained in Step 1 as the whole number of the mixed fraction:
>
> $$\text{Whole number} = \text{Step 1 whole number} = 1$$
>
> **Step 3:** Use the remainder (R) obtained in Step 1 as the numerator of the new fraction; use the original denominator as the new denominator:
>
> $$\text{Fraction} = \frac{\text{Step 1 remainder}}{\text{Original denominator}} = \frac{3}{5} = \frac{3}{5}$$

Step 4: Put the whole number and the fraction together to get the mixed number:

$$1 \quad \text{and} \quad \tfrac{3}{5} = 1\tfrac{3}{5}$$

Thus, the improper fraction $\tfrac{8}{5}$ is the same as the mixed number $1\tfrac{3}{5}$.

EXERCISES

3. Convert the improper fractions to mixed numbers:

a. $\tfrac{28}{4}$ = _____   f. $\tfrac{11}{6}$ = _____

b. $\tfrac{5}{2}$ = _____   g. $\tfrac{50}{13}$ = _____

c. $\tfrac{10}{3}$ = _____   h. $\tfrac{29}{9}$ = _____

d. $\tfrac{25}{2}$ = _____   i. $\tfrac{14}{5}$ = _____

e. $\tfrac{6}{2}$ = _____   j. $\tfrac{35}{7}$ = _____

☞ In exercise (**a**) the number comes out as the whole number 7. Thus the answer as a mixed number is $7\tfrac{0}{4}$. The fraction is equal to 0 so it is dropped.

4. Change the mixed numbers to improper fractions:

a. $1\tfrac{1}{3}$ = _____   f. $5\tfrac{1}{4}$ = _____

b. $10\tfrac{4}{5}$ = _____   g. $6\tfrac{12}{13}$ = _____

c. $5\tfrac{1}{20}$ = _____   h. $100\tfrac{5}{6}$ = _____

d. $4\tfrac{3}{4}$ = _____   i. $21\tfrac{1}{3}$ = _____

e. $7\tfrac{2}{7}$ = _____   j. $3\tfrac{99}{100}$ = _____

If you multiply or divide the numerator and the denominator of a fraction by the same nonzero number, you get an *equivalent fraction*.

Example

$$\frac{3}{4} = \frac{3 \times 2}{4 \times 2} = \frac{6}{8}$$

$$\frac{6}{8} = \frac{6 \div 2}{8 \div 2} = \frac{3}{4}$$

Thus, $\tfrac{3}{4}$ and $\tfrac{6}{8}$ are equivalent fractions.

EXERCISES

5. Change each fraction to an equivalent fraction:

a. $\frac{1}{5} = \frac{?}{15}$? = _____

d. $\frac{5}{6} = \frac{?}{30}$? = _____

b. $\frac{2}{3} = \frac{?}{6}$? = _____

e. $\frac{1}{12} = \frac{?}{48}$? = _____

c. $\frac{3}{4} = \frac{?}{16}$? = _____

f. $\frac{3}{8} = \frac{?}{64}$? = _____

A fraction is in its *lowest terms* when no nonzero number except 1 can be evenly divided into both the numerator and the denominator.

Example

$$\frac{10 \div 2}{12 \div 2} = \frac{5}{6}$$

Thus, 5/6 is 10/12 reduced to its lowest terms.

EXERCISES

6. Find the lowest terms of the following fractions:

a. $\frac{2}{6}$ = _____

f. $\frac{25}{100}$ = _____

b. $\frac{3}{12}$ = _____

g. $\frac{3}{27}$ = _____

c. $\frac{4}{16}$ = _____

h. $\frac{40}{64}$ = _____

d. $\frac{3}{21}$ = _____

i. $\frac{15}{45}$ = _____

e. $\frac{8}{56}$ = _____

j. $\frac{100}{400}$ = _____

Addition and Subtraction of Fractions

To add (or subtract) fractions whose denominators are the same, just add (or subtract) the numerators and keep the denominator the same.

Example

$$\frac{2}{5} + \frac{1}{5} = \frac{2+1}{5} = \frac{3}{5} \qquad \frac{2}{5} - \frac{1}{5} = \frac{2-1}{5} = \frac{1}{5}$$

To add (or subtract) fractions whose denominators are not the same, first convert the fractions to equivalent fractions with the lowest common denominator, then add (or subtract) the numerators.

Example

Find the lowest common denominator of $\frac{1}{2}$ and $\frac{1}{3}$. The lowest number divisible by 2 and 3 is 6, so 6 is the lowest common denominator. Now change the fractions to equivalent fractions using 6 as the new denominator:

$$\frac{1}{2} = \frac{1 \times 3}{2 \times 3} = \frac{3}{6}$$

$$\frac{1}{3} = \frac{1 \times 2}{3 \times 2} = \frac{2}{6}$$

Example

$$\frac{1}{2} + \frac{1}{3} = \frac{3}{6} + \frac{2}{6} = \frac{5}{6}$$

$$\frac{1}{2} - \frac{1}{3} = \frac{3}{6} - \frac{2}{6} = \frac{1}{6}$$

$$\frac{3}{4} + \frac{1}{8} = \frac{6}{8} + \frac{1}{8} = \frac{7}{8}$$

EXERCISES

7. Add or subtract the following fractions.

		Lowest Common Denominator	Equivalent Fractions $\frac{7}{12} + \frac{2}{12}$	Result $\frac{9}{12}$	Lowest Terms $\frac{3}{4}$
a.	$\frac{7}{12} + \frac{1}{6}$ =	12			
b.	$\frac{2}{3} + \frac{1}{9}$ =				
c.	$\frac{1}{4} + \frac{1}{3}$ =				
d.	$\frac{5}{8} + \frac{1}{24}$ =				
e.	$\frac{1}{4} + \frac{1}{5}$ =				
f.	$\frac{5}{8} - \frac{1}{4}$ =				
g.	$\frac{8}{9} - \frac{2}{3}$ =				
h.	$\frac{7}{25} - \frac{1}{5}$ =				

To add (or subtract) mixed numbers, convert the mixed numbers to improper fractions, find the lowest common denominator, then add (or subtract) as usual.

Example

$$4\tfrac{2}{3}+1\tfrac{1}{6}=\frac{14}{3}+\frac{7}{6}=\frac{28}{6}+\frac{7}{6}=\frac{35}{6}=5\tfrac{5}{6}$$

$$6\tfrac{3}{4}-2\tfrac{1}{3}=\frac{27}{4}-\frac{7}{3}=\frac{81}{12}-\frac{28}{12}=\frac{53}{12}=4\tfrac{5}{12}$$

EXERCISES

8. Add or subtract the following mixed numbers:

a. $4\tfrac{1}{4}+2\tfrac{7}{8}$ = _____

b. $10+5\tfrac{1}{5}$ = _____

c. $12\tfrac{1}{16}+2\tfrac{3}{32}$ = _____

d. $6-3\tfrac{1}{2}$ = _____

e. $4\tfrac{2}{3}-1\tfrac{1}{4}$ = _____

f. $13\tfrac{5}{8}-11$ = _____

g. $5\tfrac{1}{3}+3\tfrac{2}{9}$ = _____

h. $20\tfrac{11}{15}-\tfrac{1}{5}$ = _____

i. $17-\tfrac{15}{16}$ = _____

j. $60+2\tfrac{1}{7}$ = _____

Multiplication and Division of Fractions

To multiply two fractions, multiply the numerators by the numerators and the denominators by the denominators. Always reduce the result to lowest terms.

Example

$$\frac{2}{3}\times\frac{1}{4}=\frac{2\times1}{3\times4}=\frac{2}{12}=\frac{1}{6}$$

To divide two fractions, invert the divisor, then multiply.

Example

$$\frac{1}{5}\div\frac{3}{8}=\frac{1}{5}\times\frac{8}{3}=\frac{8}{15}$$

To multiply or divide mixed numbers, first convert them into improper fractions, then multiply or divide.

Example

$$1\tfrac{1}{4} \times 2\tfrac{1}{8} = \frac{5}{4} \times \frac{17}{8}$$

$$= \frac{85}{32}$$

$$= 2\tfrac{21}{32}$$

$$2\tfrac{1}{2} \div 3\tfrac{1}{3} = \frac{5}{2} \div \frac{10}{3}$$

$$= \frac{5}{2} \times \frac{3}{10}$$

$$= \frac{15}{20}$$

$$= \frac{3}{4}$$

EXERCISES

9. Multiply or divide the following fractions:

a. $\frac{9}{20} \times \frac{3}{4}$ = _____

b. $\frac{5}{8} \times \frac{2}{3}$ = _____

c. $1\tfrac{1}{2} \times 5\tfrac{2}{3}$ = _____

d. $\frac{1}{3} \times 1\tfrac{1}{6}$ = _____

e. $3\tfrac{1}{2} \div 1\tfrac{2}{3}$ = _____

f. $1\tfrac{5}{6} \div 2$ = _____

g. $2\tfrac{1}{2} \div 3\tfrac{1}{3}$ = _____

h. $3 \div \tfrac{1}{4}$ = _____

i. $\frac{3}{16} \times \frac{2}{3}$ = _____

j. $\frac{1}{10} \times 100$ = _____

k. $\frac{1}{7} \div \frac{2}{7}$ = _____

l. $\frac{1}{64} \div \frac{1}{8}$ = _____

10. Liu has 50 cc of lidocaine and two syringes on her back table. The doctor needs $\frac{1}{2}$ of this solution to inject into the chin and $\frac{1}{4}$ of the solution to inject into the earlobe. How much of the lidocaine should Liu draw up into each syringe?
Hint: $\frac{1}{2}$ of the solution is the same as $\frac{1}{2}$ *times* the solution.

11. Trini has 1000 cubic centimeters of solution in a pitcher. One-eighth of the solution is antibiotic A and $\frac{1}{8}$ of the solution is antibiotic B. How many cubic centimeters of the solution are represented by antibiotics?

12. The patient's defect was $3\tfrac{1}{8}$ inches long and $2\tfrac{1}{5}$ inches wide. Doctor Martinez took a skin graft from the patient's right thigh, which was

$4\frac{1}{2}$ inches long and $2\frac{1}{2}$ inches wide. How much of the graft's length and width will be left over after it is used to fill the defect?

13. The laceration was $5\frac{1}{16}$ inches long. It was cleaned and a Telfa dressing was applied. If the Telfa extended $\frac{1}{4}$ inch past the laceration on each end, how long was the Telfa?

14. Susie worked overtime every day last week:

Monday $8\frac{1}{2}$ hours
Tuesday $9\frac{1}{4}$ hours
Wednesday $8\frac{3}{4}$ hours
Thursday 10 hours
Friday $8\frac{1}{4}$ hours

If overtime is anything over 40 hours in a week, how much overtime did Susie have?

Decimals

Decimal numbers are written by placing digits (0, 1, 2, 3, 4, 5, 6, 7, 8, 9) into place value columns that are separated by a **decimal point,** as shown in Table 1–2. The *place value columns* are read in sequence from left to right as multiples of decreasing powers of 10:

- Numbers to the *left* of the decimal point represent values *greater than* 1.
- Numbers to the *right* of the decimal point represent values *less than* 1.
- The number sequence is added.

**Decimal
Point**

| hundreds | tens | ones | | tenths | hundredths | thousandths |

$652.345 = (6 \times 100) + (5 \times 10) + (2 \times 1) \bullet (3 \times 1/10) + (4 \times 1/100) + (5 \times 1/1000)$

$\quad\quad\quad 600 \;+\; 50 \;+\; 2 \;\bullet\; 3/10 \;+\; 4/100 \;+\; 5/1000$

☞ Notice that each place value is a power of 10:

$652.345 = (6 \times 10^2) + (5 \times 10^1) + (2 \times 10^0) + (3 \times 10^{-1}) + (4 \times 10^{-2}) + (5 \times 10^{-3})$
$\quad\quad\quad = (6 \times 100) + (5 \times 10) + (2 \times 1) + (3 \times 1/10) + (4 \times 1/100) + (5 \times 1/1000)$

Remember:

$10^2 = 10 \times 10$
$10^1 = 10$
$10^0 = 1$
$10^{-1} = 1/10$
$10^{-2} = 1/100$

TABLE 1–2 Decimal Place Values

ten thousands	thousands	hundreds	tens	ones	decimal point	tenths	hundredths	thousandths	ten thousandths	hundred thousandths	millionths	or			
												Ten thousands	10,000.	=	10^4
												Thousands	1,000.	=	10^3
												Hundreds	100.	=	10^2
												Tens	10.	=	10^1
												Ones	1.	=	10^0
												Decimal point	.		
												Tenths	.1	=	10^{-1}
												Hundredths	.01	=	10^{-2}
												Thousandths	.001	=	10^{-3}
												Ten-thousandths	.000 1	=	10^{-4}
												Hundred-thousandths	.000 01	=	10^{-5}
												Millionths	.000 001	=	10^{-6}
10^4	10^3	10^2	10^1	10^0	•	10^{-1}	10^{-2}	10^{-3}	10^{-4}	10^{-5}	10^{-6}				

The decimal 652.345 can be read as "six hundred fifty-two point three four five." It can also be read as "six hundred fifty-two *and* three hundred forty-five thousand**ths**." Notice that

- the word "and" is used for the decimal point
- the decimal fraction is named for the rightmost place in the place column sequence
- the suffix **-th** is used to signify fractions

Example

5.45 is read as five "and" forty-five hundredths.

EXERCISES

15. Write the following in decimal form:

a. Five and five tenths = _____

b. Ten and one thousandths = _____

c. Four hundred twenty-five and three hundred three thousandths = _____

    d. One hundred fifty and fifty-seven millionths = _____

    e. Three thousand and thirty-five hundredths = _____

16. Write the following decimals in words.

    a. 951.03   = _____

    b. 1994.251 = _____

    c. 274.10   = _____

    d. 333.333 = _____

    e. 15.0045 = _____

Addition and Subtraction of Decimals

To add or subtract decimal numbers, line up the decimal points and carry out the calculations.

Example

$24.531 + 2.798 =$

         — Align the decimal points

    24.531
     2.798
    27.329

$5.04 - 1.213 =$

     5.040 ← Add zero as a place holder
   −1.213
    3.827

EXERCISES

17. Add or subtract the following decimals. [*Hint:* Add zeros as place holders.]

    a. 2.92 + 3.82   = _____

    b. 7.89 + 0.3   = _____

c. $7.56 + 1.520$ = _____

d. $0.082 + 1.5$ = _____

e. $6.354 + 4.453$ = _____

f.   5.132   g. $7.50   h.   3.009

        1.82 $ .25   2.51

     + 1.9   + $3.10   + 4.2

i. $94.35 - 84.21$ = _____

j. $2.5 - 1.321$ = _____

k. $50.20 - 25.7$ = _____

l. $8 - 5.476$ = _____

m. $46 - 0.0078$ = _____

n. $565.511 - 123.35$ = _____

Multiplication and Division of Decimals

To multiply two decimals, carry out the multiplication, then add the number of decimal places from the right of the decimal point in the original two numbers. This total is the number of decimal places from the right of the decimal point in the product.

Example

    0.07   2 decimal places

   × 2.1   +1 decimal place

    007

    014

  0.147   3 decimal places

  .00051   5 decimal places

   × .04   + 2 decimal places

.0000204   7 decimal places

   └─┘ —————————— Add zeros

To divide decimals by whole numbers, carry out the long division. Align the decimal point of the quotient directly above that of the dividend.

Example

Align decimal points in
quotient and dividend

$$
\begin{array}{r}
3.09 \\
5\overline{)15.45} \\
\underline{15} \\
45 \\
\underline{45} \\
0
\end{array}
$$

If the divisor is a decimal, convert it to a whole number before dividing. To do this, move the decimal point of the divisor and that of the dividend the same number of places to the right.

Example

$$
2.5\overline{)6.25} \quad = \quad 2\underset{\smile}{.}5\overline{)6\underset{\smile}{.}2.5}
$$

$$
\begin{array}{r}
2.5 \\
\underline{50} \\
125 \\
\underline{125} \\
0
\end{array}
$$

One place
value

Divisor ———→ ⌐⌐ ←——— Whole number

(1) 2.5 × 10 = 25
(2) 6.25 × 10 = 62.5

Dividend ———↑

Two place
values

Divisor ———→ ⌐⌐ ←——— Whole number

$$
.25\overline{)5} \quad = \quad \underset{\smile}{.}25\overline{)5\underset{\smile}{.}00\underset{\smile}{.}}
$$

$$
\begin{array}{r}
20. \\
\underline{50} \\
00
\end{array}
$$

(1) .25 × 100 = 25
(2) 5 × 100 = 500

Dividend ———↑

EXERCISES

18. Multiply the following decimals:

a. 5 × .04   = _____

b. 12 × .3   = _____

c. 100 × .07 = _____

d. $.12 \times .5 \quad =$ _____

e. $1.3 \times .9 \quad =$ _____

19. Divide the following decimals:

a. $.8 \div 2 \qquad =$ _____

b. $15 \div .3 \qquad =$ _____

c. $.120 \div .40 \quad =$ _____

d. $54.63 \div .9 \quad =$ _____

e. $101.53 \div .71 =$ _____

When more than one operation (addition, subtraction, multiplication, division) must be carried out, use the *order of operations:*

Parentheses
Multiplication
Division
Addition
Subtraction

Example

$4 + 5(4 + 3) =$	$(4 + 5) + (4 + 3) =$	$4 + (5 + 4)3 =$
$4 + 5(7) \quad =$	$9 \quad + \quad 7 \quad = 16$	$4 + \quad (9)3 \quad =$
$4 + 35 \quad = 39$		$4 + \quad 27 \quad = 31$

To convert fractions to decimals, divide the numerator by the denominator.

Example

$$\frac{1}{4} = 4\overline{)1.00} \quad \begin{array}{r} .25 \\ \underline{8} \\ 20 \\ \underline{20} \\ 0 \end{array}$$

$$\frac{2}{3} = 3\overline{)2.0000} \quad \begin{array}{r} .666... \\ \underline{1\,8} \\ 20 \\ \underline{18} \\ 20 \end{array} \quad = .\overline{66}$$

☞ When the answer is a nonterminating number, you may signify this with a line over the repeating numerals.

EXERCISES

20. Multiply or divide the following decimals.

a. $.02 \times .02$ = _____

b. 3.1×3 = _____

c. $100 \times .04$ = _____

d. 6.22×5.4 = _____

e. $.0007 \times .08$ = _____

f. $35.96 \div 5.8$ = _____

g. $1.001 \div .13$ = _____

h. $6.4 \div .08$ = _____

i. $.324 \div .09$ = _____

j. $.005 \div 2.5$ = _____

To convert decimals to fractions, the decimal numeral expressed becomes the numerator and the decimal place (tenths, hundredths) becomes the denominator.

Example

.95   95 is the decimal expressed and becomes the numerator 1/100 or hundredths is the decimal place expressed and so becomes the denominator

thus, $.95 = \frac{95}{100}$

☞ To round to the nearest tenth, carry the division out to the next decimal value after tenths (hundredths). If this number is 5 or greater, round the number in tenths place up. If this number is less than 5, the number in tenths place remains the same.

EXERCISES

21. Convert the fractions into decimals (rounded to the nearest thousandth).

a. $\frac{1}{3}$ = _____

b. $\frac{5}{8}$ = _____

c. $\frac{3}{4}$ = _____

d. $\frac{11}{16}$ = _____

e. $\frac{7}{30}$ = _____

f. $\frac{8}{64}$ = _____

g. $\frac{2}{9}$ = _____

h. $\frac{3}{100}$ = _____

i. $\frac{3}{15}$ = _____

j. $\frac{6}{8}$ = _____

22. Convert the decimals to fractions and reduce to lowest terms.

a. $.003$ = _____

b. $.5$ = _____

c. $.75$ = _____

d. $.90$ = _____

e. $.051$ = _____

23. One inch is equal to 2.54 centimeters. The doctor wishes to take a 3-inch long by 2-inch wide skin graft from the donor site. How many centimeters long will this graft be?

24. The silastic block for implantation was 4 inches thick. The doctor used 1.44 inches of its thickness on his first case. How many inches thick was the leftover silastic block?

25. The surgical technologist made $74.10 for 6.5 hours of work. How much did the technologist make each hour?

26. A medicine is given by the anesthesiologist according to the patient's weight in kilograms. For every kilogram, $\frac{1}{4}$ cc of the medicine is needed. If the patient weighs 110 pounds and there are 2.2 pounds per kilogram, how much of the medicine will be needed?

27. Dr. Ho drilled a hole in the femur. The hole was 2.68 centimeters deep. The shortest screw in the set was 2.75 centimeters. How much longer than the hole was the screw?

Percentages

Percents are special types of fractions which mean "per every hundred." Thus the denominator of a percent is always understood to be 100 and is shown by the symbol % rather than being written.

A percent can be written as a fraction by putting the number expressed as the numerator and the denominator as 100. It can be written as a decimal by putting down the number expressed and moving the decimal point two places to the left, thus signifying hundredths.

Example

$25\% = \frac{25}{100}$ or $\frac{1}{4}$

$25\% = .25$

In other words, when you drop the % sign, either replace it with a denominator of 100 or a decimal place of hundredths. When you add the % sign, either drop the denominator of 100 or move the decimal point two places to the right.

EXERCISES

28. Convert the following percents to fractions and then decimals:

a. 5% = _____ and _____

b. 51% = _____ and _____

c. 1% = _____ and _____

29. Complete the following table:

percent	fraction	decimal
a. _____	$\frac{3}{4}$	_____
b. 10%	_____	_____
c. _____	_____	.3
d. _____	$\frac{3}{8}$	_____
e. 60%	_____	_____

To find the percent of a number, change the percent to a decimal or fraction, replace the "of" with the times ($\times$) sign, and multiply.

Example

10% of 100 =

$.10 \times 100 = 10$ or $\frac{10}{100}$, which is reduced to $\frac{1}{10} \times 100 = 10$

To find what percent one number is of another, make the numbers into a fraction with the number following the "of" as the denominator. Then convert the fraction into a decimal and then into a percent.

Example

(1) 9 is what percent of 27?
$\frac{9}{27} = \frac{1}{3} = .333$ or 33.3%

(2) 5 is what percent of 25?
$\frac{5}{25} = \frac{1}{5} = .20 = 20\%$

EXERCISES

30. Solve the following.

a. 3 is what percent of 30? _____

b. 15 is what percent of 75? _____

c. 40 is what percent of 80? _____

Table 1–3 Common Fractions, Decimals, and Percents

Fraction	Decimal	Percent
1/2	0.5	50%
1/4	0.25	25%
3/4	0.75	75%
1/3	0.333*	33 1/3%
2/3	0.666*	66 2/3%
1/5	0.2	20%
2/5	0.4	40%
3/5	0.6	60%
4/5	0.8	80%
1/10	0.1	10%
1/1	1.0	100%

* 0.333 and 0.666 are *nonterminating* decimals. This means the number patterns .333 . . . and .666 . . . go on forever.

   d. 2 is what percent of 100? _____

   e. What percent of 25 is 20? _____

31. On the final exam, Alice left 10% of the questions blank. If there were 50 questions, how many did she leave unanswered?

32. The work schedule for each surgical employee is made out for 30 days of work per rotation. Calvin missed 5% of his work days during the last schedule. How many days did Calvin actually work?

33. The patient weighed 180 pounds. During surgery, a 9-pound tumor was removed from the patient's abdomen. What percent of the patient's total preoperative weight was actually tumor?

34. The surgical technology students spent 10% of their clinical hours in Labor and Delivery and 15% of their clinical hours in Central Supply. If their clinical hours totaled 1020, how many hours were spent in Labor and Delivery? In Central Supply?

Refer to Table 1–3 for equivalent values of the more commonly used fractions, decimals, and percents.

Ratio and Proportion

A **ratio** is a comparison of two numbers, *a* and *b*, expressed as

$$a:b \quad \text{or} \quad a/b \quad \text{or} \quad \frac{a}{b}$$

Example

A two-to-one ratio is expressed as

$$2:1 \quad \text{or} \quad 2/1 \quad \text{or} \quad \frac{2}{1}$$

A **proportion** is a statement of equality between ratios: $a/b = c/d$ or $a:b = c:d$

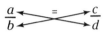 where a and d are the *extremes*
and b and c are the *means*

or

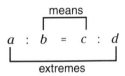

In any proportion, the product of the means must equal the product of the extremes: $a \times d = b \times c$

Example

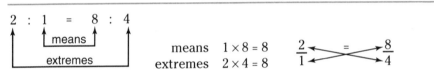

Proportions can be used to solve for an unknown term when the other three terms are known. Let x be the unknown. Set up the proportion, multiply the means and the extremes, and solve for x.

Example

Given $2:3 = x:9$, what is x?

$\dfrac{2}{3} = \dfrac{x}{9}$ \quad Set up the proportion

$3x = 2 \times 9$ \quad Multiply the means and extremes

$3x = 18$

$x = 18/3$ \quad Divide by the coefficient of x

$\quad = 6$

EXERCISES

35. Solve for the unknown (x) in the following proportions:

a. $2:10 = 16:x$ $x =$ _____

b. $7:30 = x:90$ $x =$ _____

c. $2.5:5 = x:50$ $x =$ _____

d. $16:x = 24:3$ $x =$ _____

e. $5:300 = 10:x$ $x =$ _____

You can use ratios and proportion to calculate the quantities of drugs. To do this, you need to know that *strength* is a ratio—it is always expressed as units of one substance **per** unit or units of another substance. Sometimes we express strength as weight per unit of volume—e.g., the strength of Demerol may be 100 mg (milligrams) of Demerol per 1 mL (milliliter) of solution. And sometimes we express strength per hundred units of another substance. For example a 5% saline solution is 5 grams of sodium chloride NaCl per 100 grams of water.

☞   1 cubic centimeter (cc) of water weighs 1 gram, so a 5% solution of saline is also 5 grams per cubic centimeter (gm/cc)

Example

The doctor has prescribed 50 milligrams of Demerol. The Demerol solution you have on the back table has a strength of 100 milligrams per milliliter (mg/mL). How many milliliters of that solution do you need?

   This relationship is a proportion, $100:1 = 50:x$, or

$$\frac{100 \text{ milligrams}}{1 \text{ milliliter}} = \frac{50 \text{ milligrams}}{x \text{ milliliters}}$$

Multiplying the means and extremes, $100 \times x = 50 \times 1$, you get

$$100x = 50$$
$$x = 50/100$$
$$= .5 = 1/2 \text{ mL}$$

Sometimes we can think of ratios in terms of parts of a whole. In this case, it's easy to think about percents.

Example

You want to make up a 3:3:4 solution of saline, Lincocin, and Garamycin. (**a**) What percentage of the solution does each ingredient represent? (**b**) If you wanted to make up 200 milliliters of this solution, how many milliliters of saline would you use? Lincocin? Garamycin?

(**a**) 3:3:4 means three parts to three parts to four parts. That is, you need a total of

$$3 + 3 + 4 = 10 \text{ parts in the whole solution}$$

By convention, the parts are listed in the same order as ingredients, so you have

3 parts of saline in 10 parts of solution $= 3/10 = 30/100 = .3 = 30\%$
3 parts of Lincocin in 10 parts of solution $= 3/10 = 30/100 = .3 = 30\%$
4 parts of Garamycin in 10 parts of solution $= 4/10 = 40/100 = .4 = 40\%$

(**b**) You want 200 mL of solution, so you multiply each ingredient's percentage by 200:

Saline (30%):　　　　$.30 \times 200$ milliliters $=\ 60$ milliliters
Lincocin (30%):　　　$.30 \times 200$ milliliters $=\ 60$ milliliters
Garamycin (40%):　　$.40 \times 200$ milliliters $=\ \underline{80}$ milliliters
TOTAL　　　　　　　　　　　　　　　　　　　　　$\overline{200}$ milliliters

To calculate a dilution, you can use the *standard dilution equation:*

$$C_1 \times V_1 = C_2 \times V_2$$

where C stands for concentration in (percent) and V stands for volume. Thus

$C_1 = $ Concentration 1
$C_2 = $ Concentration 2
$V_1 = $ Volume 1
$V_2 = $ Volume 2

Example

The procedure calls for 60 cubic centimeters (cc) of 1/2% dye. How much saline and how much 1% dye solution do you need to make up the required amount of solution?

Here, you're being asked for a dilution, so you start by sorting out what you know from what you don't know:

$C_1 = 1/2 = .5\%$　　Concentration 1　　KNOWN (asked for)
$C_2 = 1 \%$　　　　　Concentration 2　　KNOWN (given)
$V_1 = 60$　　　　　　Volume 1　　　　　KNOWN (asked for)
$V_2 = x$　　　　　　Volume 2　　　　　UNKNOWN volume of saline

Now you can write the standard dilution equation as

$$C_1 \times V_1 = C_2 \times V_2$$
$$1/2 \times 60 = 1 \times x$$
$$30 = x$$
$$x = 30 \text{ cc of saline}$$

So you add $x = 30$ cc of pure saline to $60 - x = 30$ cc of 1% dye solution to get 60 cc of .5% dye solution.

EXERCISES

36. The procedure calls for 60 cc of 1/2% radiopaque dye. You have 1% dye. How much sterile saline and how much 1% dye should you use to make the proper amount of the needed solution?

37. Doctor Rojas wants 1/2% Ponticaine solution for her procedure. You have 25 cc of 1% Ponticaine. How do you dilute it to the proper strength?

38. What percent of saline is present in a 2:3 mixture of tincture and saline?

39. Doctor Smith wants 1/2% Xylocaine solution for his procedure. You have 50 cc of 1% Xylocaine. How do you dilute it to the proper strength?

40. Doctor Smith from the problem above wants to use 1/4 of the solution on the face and 1/2 of the solution on the neck. How much of the solution should you draw up for each area?

41. You have a 4:5:1 solution of water, alcohol, and tincture. What percent of the solution does each ingredient represent?

42. The order calls for a dosage of 20 milligrams of a medicine that comes in a concentration of 4 milligrams per 1 milliliter. How many milliliters will you need?

43. The doctor's preference card calls for 300 milligrams of antibiotic A to be added to the 1000 milliliters of irrigation solution in your pitcher on the back table. Antibiotic A comes in a concentration of 10 milligrams per 2 milliliters. How many milliliters of the antibiotic should you add to your pitcher?

44. Acetaminophen 650 milligrams is prescribed. The medicine is available as 325-milligram tablets. To give 650 milligrams, how many tablets would be needed?

Note: Try using the formula

$$\frac{D}{H} = \frac{x}{V}$$

where D = desired dose (dose ordered), H = dose on hand, V = unit (one tablet here), and x is the unknown number of tablets.

Temperature Conversions

In medicine we use two scales to measure temperature (see Fig. 1–1): the **Fahrenheit scale** and the **Celsius** (centigrade) **scale.** In the Fahrenheit scale, the boiling point of water is 212°F and its freezing point is 32°F. In the Celsius scale, the boiling point of water at 100°C and its freezing point is 0°C. Nine degrees on the Fahrenheit scale corresponds to 5 degrees on the Celsius scale. Using these ratios, the following formulas (see Table 1–4) were developed to convert temperatures from one scale to the other.

$$C = 5/9 \ (F - 32)$$
$$F = 9/5 \ C + 32$$

where C is the Celsius temperature and F is the Fahrenheit temperature.

Temperature is important in many aspects of the surgical setting, and readings may be given in Fahrenheit or Celsius degrees. The surgical patient's body temperature is of vital importance and is constantly monitored. Normal body

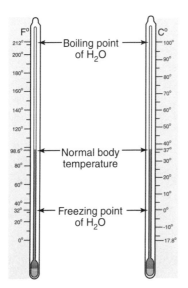

Figure 1–1 Fahrenheit and Celsius Scales.

Table 1–4 Temperature Conversions

To Convert from	Use the Formula	The Operation Means
Fahrenheit to Celsius	$C = \frac{5}{9}(F - 32)$	(1) Subtract 32 from the Fahrenheit temperature (2) Multiply this number by $\frac{5}{9}$
Celsius to Fahrenheit	$F = \frac{9}{5}C + 32$	(1) Multiply the Celsius temperature by $\frac{9}{5}$ (2) Add 32 to the result

temperature is 98.6°F or 37°C. Preoperatively, an elevated temperature could signify an infection or other health problem. This could result in the postponement of the surgical procedure. Intraoperatively, the body temperature is monitored by anesthesia personnel. An abnormal body temperature—whether below normal (*hypothermia*) or elevated (*hyperthermia*)—alters the basal metabolic rate, interfering with blood pressure, heart rate, circulation, etc. Hyperthermia can also indicate life-threatening situations such as malignant hyperthermia (see Chapter 15). Postoperatively, temperature is monitored for the same reasons, and an elevated temperature at this time may indicate a wound infection. Another surgical aspect of temperature is the sterilization of instruments and equipment. Here, temperature along with pressure and time is monitored for proper sterilization. Temperature is also important for the surgical environment. Each surgical room is kept at 68° to 75°F (20° to 24°C) to discourage the growth of bacteria that can cause surgical wound infections. It is also important to keep the room at this temperature range for the comfort of surgical personnel who are working under surgical lights attired in full scrub apparel. A cool environment decreases the chance that perspiration will drip from a surgical team member onto the sterile field.

EXERCISES

45. Convert the following (round to the nearest tenth):

    a. 120°F = _____°C

    b. 120°C = _____°F

    c. 86°F = _____°C

    d. 185°C = _____°F

    e. 98.6°F = _____°C

    f. 270°F = _____°C

Measurement Systems

While the surgical technologist does not routinely administer medication directly to the patient, the technologist is responsible for obtaining medicines and mixing them for use in the sterile field. You may, for example, have to mix antibiotics in an irrigation solution. This may require you to convert from one measurement system to another. Therefore, you'll need to know conversion equivalents and be able to perform the calculations involved in such conversions.

There are three measurement systems commonly used in medicine. They are the metric, apothecary, and household systems.

The Metric System

The **metric system** is the *international standard* (used by scientists and engineers everywhere) of weights and measures. Developed by the French in the eighteenth century, it has been adopted by most European countries as their common measurement system. (Eventually, the metric system will be used exclusively by everyone.) It is also utilized extensively in the health care field. The *United States Pharmacopoeia,* for example, uses it exclusively and all specimens sent to pathology are weighed and measured in metric terms. The metric system allows a way to calculate small drug dosages, and most manufacturers use this system for calibration in the development of new drugs. Most medications used in surgery are dispensed utilizing the metric system of measurement.

In the metric system, length, volume, and weight (mass) are measured against certain defined units called *base units:*

Length—the *meter* (m)
Volume—the *liter* (L)
Weight—the *gram* (g)

Each of these base units is divided into smaller and larger units based on multiples of 10, and these multiples are indicated by prefixes:

Prefix (abbreviation)	Multiply base unit by . . .
micro (μ)	.000001 (or 1/1,000,000)
milli (m)	.001 (or 1/1000)
centi (c)	.01 (or 1/100)
deci (d)	.1 (or 1/10)
UNIT	meter, liter, gram
deka (da)	10.
hecto (h)	100.
kilo (k)	1000.

Any prefix can be used with any base unit to indicate a measurement. For example, 1 **m**m = .001 m, 1 **m**L = .001 L, and 1 **m**g = .001 g; similarly, 1 **k**m = 1000 m, 1 **k**L = 1000 L, and 1 **k**g = 1000 g. But you'll be most concerned with just a few of them—particularly, micro, milli, and centi.

Because the metric system is based on the decimal system, conversions are very easy. You just have to recognize the correct multiple of 10. Then you can use the appropriate unit conversion.

Unit Conversion		
Length		
1 meter = 1000 millimeters	$\frac{1 \text{ m}}{1000 \text{ mm}} = 1$ or	$\frac{1000 \text{ mm}}{1 \text{ m}} = 1$
1 meter = 100 centimeters	$\frac{1 \text{ m}}{100 \text{ cm}} = 1$ or	$\frac{100 \text{ cm}}{1 \text{ m}} = 1$
1 meter = 1,000,000 micrometers (microns)	$\frac{1 \text{ m}}{1,000,000 \text{ μm}} = 1$ or	$\frac{1,000,000 \text{ μm}}{1 \text{ m}} = 1$
1 millimeter = 1000 micrometers (microns)	$\frac{1 \text{ mm}}{1000 \text{ μm}} = 1$ or	$\frac{1000 \text{ μm}}{1 \text{ mm}} = 1$
Volume		
1 liter = 1000 milliliters	$\frac{1 \text{ L}}{1000 \text{ mL}} = 1$ or	$\frac{1000 \text{ mL}}{1 \text{ L}} = 1$
1 kiloliter = 1000 liters	$\frac{1 \text{ kL}}{1000 \text{ L}} = 1$ or	$\frac{1000 \text{ L}}{1 \text{ kL}} = 1$
Weight (mass)		
1 gram = 1000 milligrams	$\frac{1 \text{ g}}{1000 \text{ mg}} = 1$ or	$\frac{1000 \text{ mg}}{1 \text{ g}} = 1$
1 gram = 1,000,000 micrograms	$\frac{1 \text{ g}}{1,000,000 \text{ μg}} = 1$ or	$\frac{1,000,000 \text{ μg}}{1 \text{ g}} = 1$
1 milligram = 1000 micrograms	$\frac{1 \text{ mg}}{1000 \text{ μg}} = 1$ or	$\frac{1000 \text{ μg}}{1 \text{ mg}} = 1$
1 kilogram = 1000 grams	$\frac{1 \text{ kg}}{1000 \text{ g}} = 1$ or	$\frac{1000 \text{ g}}{1 \text{ kg}} = 1$

METRIC COMPARISONS

The meter is about 39.37 inches, just over a yard (36 inches). It's a linear measure used for lengths, including heights and widths. For example, patient height is measured in meters, while tumors, flaps, and defects are measured as lengths and widths—usually in centimeters or millimeters (hundredths or thousandths of meters). Note that when a length measure is multiplied by another length measure, the result is an area, which is a *square measure.* For instance, a defect that is 10 cm by 5 cm has an area of $5 \times 10 = 50$ cm^2.

The meter is related to volume by *cubic measure.* When 1 centimeter is multiplied by itself three times—1 cm $\times$ 1 cm $\times$ 1 cm—it becomes the volume 1 cubic centimeter (1 cm^3), which is about the same size as a sugar cube. When length, width, and height (or depth) are multiplied together, the result is measured in cubic terms. Thus, a block of tissue that is 5 cm long, 3 cm wide, and 1 cm deep is $5 \times 3 \times 1 = 15$ cm^3.

The liter is a fluid (or liquid) measure approximately equal to a quart (1 L = 1.06 qt). Most medicines in surgery are in liquid form, including intravenous and irrigation solutions (often measured in liters) as well as many antibiotic solutions (usually measured in milliliters or thousandths of liters). In medicine, however, we call a cm^3 a "cc" (short for cubic centimeter, of course). This liquid measure

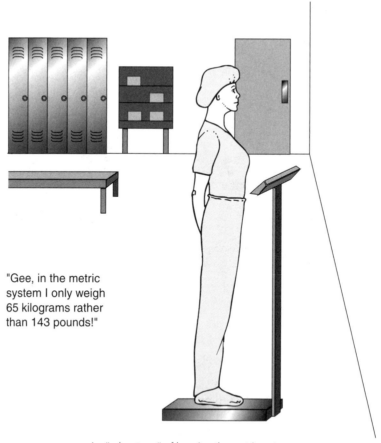

"Gee, in the metric
system I only weigh
65 kilograms rather
than 143 pounds!"

An "advantage" of learning the metric system.

of volume is related to the solid measure by one simple definition: 1 cc = 1 cm³ = 1 mL. You'll see and hear these terms used interchangeably.

The gram is a small unit of mass (or weight), which is much less than an ounce (30 g is about 1 oz). For a mental picture, consider a paper clip; it weighs about a gram. In this case it's easier to think in terms of kilograms. One kilogram is 2.2 pounds (picture a 2-lb can of coffee). It's worth knowing that 1 cc (1 mL) of water weighs 1 gram, which means that aqueous solutions measured in weight percent (g/100 g) can also be reckoned in grams per milliliter of solution. You'll encounter gram or milligram measures when working with drugs in powder form, such as antibiotics that must be reconstituted (dissolved) in water. And you'll encounter kilogram measures when calculating dosages determined by body weight.

☞ The metric system is, by far, the most important measuring system in the world—and the most important to you. It lets you measure—and calculate with—small and large quantities of any kind without having to multiply by such ill-behaved conversion factors as 12 inches per foot, 2 pints in a quart (and 4 quarts in a gallon), and 16 ounces per pound. All you have to do is multiply and divide by 10, which is mostly a matter of moving the decimal point the correct number of places in the proper direction. Eventually, you'll find yourself thinking in it. But if you aren't already used to it, you'll find it helpful to compare metric measures with common measures. If, for example, you already know how long an inch is, you can easily picture that length as about 2.5 cm. Table 1–5 lists some of the more common equivalents, giving approximate conversions.

Table 1–5   **Approximate Measurement Equivalents**

Weight	Length
1 kilogram = 2.2 pounds	1 meter = 39.37 inches = approx. 1 yard
1 gram = 15 grains	1 yard = 3 feet = 36 inches
1 ounce = 30 grams	1 inch = 2.54 centimeters
1 grain = 60 milligrams	

Volume

1 kiloliter = exactly 1000 liters
1 liter = 1 quart
1 milliliter = 1 gram = 15 minims = 1 cubic centimeter
1 fluid ounce = 8 fluid drams = 30 milliliters
1 gallon = 4 liters
1 pint = 500 milliliters
1 quart = 2 pints = 1000 milliliters
1 gallon = 4 quarts = 4000 milliliters
1 teaspoon = 60 drops
1 minim = 1 drop

The Apothecary System

The **apothecary system** was the system of weights and measures used for writing medication orders in ancient Greece and Rome, and in Europe during the Middle Ages. It is rarely used today. The apothecary system is based upon everyday items (such as the weight of a grain of wheat) and uses lowercase Roman numerals. For example, 4 grains would be written as gr. īv. Some medications continue to use this system, as do pharmacists, so it is important to recognize the basic units of measure of the apothecary system:

Volume—the *minim* (fluid)
Weight—the *grain*

A minim is approximately equal to one drop. (As drops vary according to the dropper used, this measurement is not always accurate. For accuracy, a calibrated dropper should be used.) Larger quantities are multiples of the minim:

60 minims   = 1 fluid dram
8 fluid drams = 1 fluid ounce
1 pint   = 16 fluid ounces
2 pints   = 1 quart
4 quarts   = 1 gallon

The grain was based upon the average weight of a grain of wheat. Larger quantities are multiples of the grain:

20 grains (xx) = 1 scruple
3 scruples   = 1 dram
60 grains   = 1 dram
12 ounces   = 1 pound
8 drams   = 1 ounce

Note that in the apothecary system, 12 ounces equals 1 pound rather than 16 ounces (as in avoirdupois weight).

☞ Although household measurements are used primarily for administering over-the-counter (OTC) medications—and never in surgery—it's useful to see how they compare with more accurate standard measures. (See chart below and Fig. 1–2.)

Household Conversions
1 teaspoon = 5 milliliters = 5 cubic centimeters = 1 fluid dram
1 tablespoon = 1/2 fluid ounce = 4 fluid drams = 15 milliliters = 15 cubic centimeters
2 tablespoons = 1 fluid ounce = 30 milliliters = 30 cubic centimeters

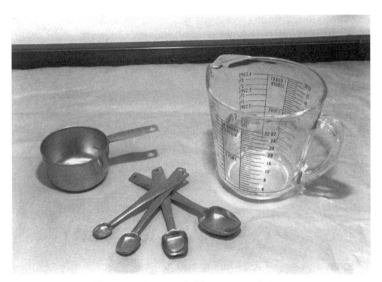

Figure 1–2 Household measuring devices.

Other Standardized Measurements (Doses)

Some medications are measured directly by their strengths— i.e., they are measured in *units* (u.) based upon their potency. A common medication measured in units is insulin. There are special insulin syringes calibrated to these units. In surgery, several antibiotics, including penicillin and Bacitracin, are also measured in units. These medications are used in antibiotic irrigation solutions during surgical procedures. Another medication measured in units is heparin, an anticoagulant administered intravenously to the patient by anesthesia personnel during vascular cases. Heparin is also used diluted in saline on the backtable.

Another measurement of medications according to their strength is the *milliequivalent* (mEq.) A milliequivalent is equal to 1/1000 (0.001) of a chemical equivalent, a measurement associated with electrolytes. Concentrations of electrolytes are often expressed as milliequivalents per liter. Electrolytes are essential for metabolic activities in the body and for normal function of body cells. A common electrolyte administered to the surgical patient is potassium chloride (KCl), which is necessary for the transmission of nerve impulses, control of heart rhythm, and fluid balance. Low potassium levels can pose a risk to the surgical patient undergoing general anesthesia. Potassium chloride is administered in milliequivalents preoperatively or by anesthesia personnel.

See Table 1–6 for a comparison of measurement systems and Table 1–7 for symbols of measurement.

Table 1–6   Comparison of Measurement Systems

The Metric System

- is used in the *United States Pharmacopoeia*
- was invented by the French in the eighteenth century
- is based upon the decimal system
- has basic units that are multiples of 10
- expresses measurements in Arabic numerals and decimals
- basic units of measure are the meter (length), liter (volume), and the gram (weight)

The Apothecary System

- is used mainly by pharmacists
- was used in ancient Greek and Roman times, then in Europe during the Middle Ages
- is based upon simple items such as a grain of wheat or a stone
- expresses measurements in Roman numerals and fractions
- basic units of measure are the minim (volume) and the grain (weight)

The Household Measuring System

- used in recipes, food products, and OTC medicines
- is easily understood by nonmedical persons
- is not accurate; should not be used in medication administration
- basic measurements include the dropper, tablespoon, teaspoon, glass, and cup

Table 1–7   Symbols of Measurement

Metric System		Apothecary System		Household System	
meter	m	minim	m, min, ɱ	teaspoon	tsp
liter	L	grain	gr	tablespoon	tbsp
cubic centimeter	cc	dram	dr, ʒ	ounce	oz
centimeter	cm	fluid dram	fl. dr, ℨ	pint	pt
millimeter	mm	drop	gtt	quart	qt
gram	g	ounce	oz	gallon	gal
kilogram	kg	pint	pt	inch	in
milligram	mg	quart	qt	yard	yd
milliliter	mL	gallon	gal		
kiloliter	kL	pound	lb		
microgram	mcg, μg	scruple	scr, ℈		
micron (micrometer)	μm				

EXERCISES

46. Convert the following:

Volume
a. 10 cc   = _____ mL

b. 1000 mL = _____ L

c. 5 gal   = _____ L

d. 1 pt   = _____ mL

e. 1 tsp   = _____ cc

Weight
f. 1 g   = _____ mg

g. 5 kg   = _____ g

h. 1 kg   = _____ lb

i. 5 lb   = _____ oz

j. 1 oz   = _____ g

Length
k. 1 m   = _____ in

l. 1 mm   = _____ μm

m. 72 in   = _____ yd

n. 1 in   = _____ cm

o. 1 cm   = _____ mm

47. Convert the following:

a. 5 min   = _____ gtt

b. 1 gr   = _____ mg

c. 15 gr   = _____ g

d. 3 tsp   = _____ gtt

e. 1/4 oz   = _____ dr

48. Write the appropriate value and abbreviations for each of the following:

a. five milliliters _____

    b. three thousandths gram _____

    c. one hundred fifty cubic centimeters _____

    d. four tenths kilogram _____

    e. one-half ounce _____

    f. seven grains _____

Summary

This chapter reviewed basic mathematical skills of addition, subtraction, multiplication, and division of fractions and decimals. Students were directed to use fractions, decimals, and percents, together with ratios and proportions, to solve problems and perform calculations and conversions. All calculations follow the order of operations and must be reduced to the lowest terms. Some of these conversions were utilized to find equivalents between measurement systems. The metric system is the most commonly used standard of weights and measures. It has been adopted by most European countries and is used in surgery. The apothecary system was the original measurement system for writing medication orders and uses Roman numerals. The household measurement system is more familiar to the nonmedical person, as it is used in recipes and over-the-counter medications. In addition to the three basic systems, other standardized measurements for specific medications were discussed. These include units (u) for insulin and milliequivalents (mEq) for electrolytes. In addition to calculations and conversions, surgical technology students must interpret accepted pharmacology language of medical symbols and abbreviations in order to properly handle and prepare medications. Equivalents of measurement between systems were presented to assist the student in making conversions.

REVIEW

1. State Roman numerals for the following:
    a. 90
    b. 150
    c. 2000

2. State Arabic numerals for the following:
    a. MMII
    b. LXVIII
    c. MDMXVI

3. Give an example of **(a)** a mixed fraction, **(b)** an improper fraction, and **(c)** an equivalent fraction.

4. What is the order of operations?

5. What is the decimal place value of 5 in .923715?

6. Complete the following statements:
a. Percents are fractions which means "per every _____".
b. In a proportion, the product of the means equals _____.

7. Which of the three basic measurement systems is preferred and why?

CHAPTER **2**

Basic Pharmacology

OBJECTIVES

Upon completion of this chapter, you should be able to:

1 Identify a contribution to the evolution of pharmacology from several eras of civilization.

2 Describe contributions to pharmacology made by key historical figures.

3 List sources of drugs and give an example of each.

4 Distinguish between generic and trade names of drugs and recognize what chemical names are.

5 List four drug classification categories and identify several subcategories in each.

6 Discuss drug orders used in surgery.

7 List the parts of a drug order.

8 Describe the drug distribution systems used in hospitals.

9 List the forms that drugs come in and recognize their abbreviations.

10 Discuss the drug administration routes used in surgery.

11 Describe the four processes of pharmacokinetics.

12 Define side effects and distinguish between adverse effects and idiosyncratic effects.

13 Recognize the abbreviations used for units of measure in basic pharmacology.

KEY TERMS

Adverse effect An undesired side effect or toxicity caused by the administration of drugs.

Agonist A drug that binds to a receptor and stimulates the receptor's function.

Antagonist A drug that counteracts the action of another drug.

Idiosyncratic effect An unusual response to a drug.

Local effect Response limited to one place or part.

Medication order A physician's request to dispense and administer a drug.

Parenteral Any medication administration route other than the alimentary canal.

Pharmacodynamics The study of drugs and their actions in living organisms.

Pharmacokinetics The study of the metabolism and action of drugs, with emphasis on the time required for absorption, duration of action, distribution in the body, and method of excretion.

Plasma protein binding The ability of drugs to attach to receptor sites on proteins contained in blood plasma.

Recombinant DNA technology (biotechnology) Artificial manipulation of segments of DNA (genetic material).

Side effect An unintended action or effect of a drug.

Solution Chemical substance(s) dissolved in water.

Suspension Undissolved chemical substance dispersed in liquid.

Systemic effect Response that affects the whole body.

The science of pharmacology is a rapidly expanding field of study, as new drugs are being developed nearly every day. An understanding of basic principles in pharmacology will help the surgical technologist deal with such constant developments. Students should endeavor to build a framework of principles, so that new information may be incorporated simply. When a new drug is introduced into surgical practice, the surgical technologist should be able to understand information about the drug by applying the principles of pharmacology. This chapter presents an introduction to the foundations of pharmacology that may be applied throughout a professional career in surgical technology.

History of Pharmacology

Illness and injury began when humankind began; therefore, the history of cures goes back to before written records. The earliest records are in the form of cave paintings, clay tablets, and papyrus scrolls. As more medical materials became known, pharmacopoeias were compiled to sort and save drug knowledge. These were formal collections of drug information and standards. The science of alchemy, which was the forerunner of later sciences, such as pharmacology and chemistry, recorded experiments and discoveries. The following provides a brief look at the development of pharmacology through the eras of civilization, as summarized in Figure 2–1.

Prehistoric Era (100,000–3000 BC [BCE])

The earliest evidence of prehistoric healing arts comes from wall paintings, rock carvings, and burial sites. At this stage, humans were primarily interested in finding food for survival. Probably, the discovery of the healing properties of roots, leaves, berries, and bark occurred accidentally as people were eating them. As much as 80,000 years ago, Paleolithic (Old Stone Age) peoples engraved drawings of plants on bones and deer antlers. A Neolithic (New Stone Age) burial site from northern Iraq revealed clusters of flowers and herbs buried with the body. When humans established larger communities, individuals took roles as healers. Part of their power came from their ability to help the sick and wounded—knowledge only the healers possessed. Primitive specialists tried to control the "spirits," which they believed were responsible for disease. These specialists eventually became priests and priestesses, sorcerers, medicine men and women, and shamans.

Ancient Era (3500–750 BC [BCE])

Ancient cultures also combined magic, religion, and rituals with drugs and healing. It was in the area between the Tigris and Euphrates river valleys near the

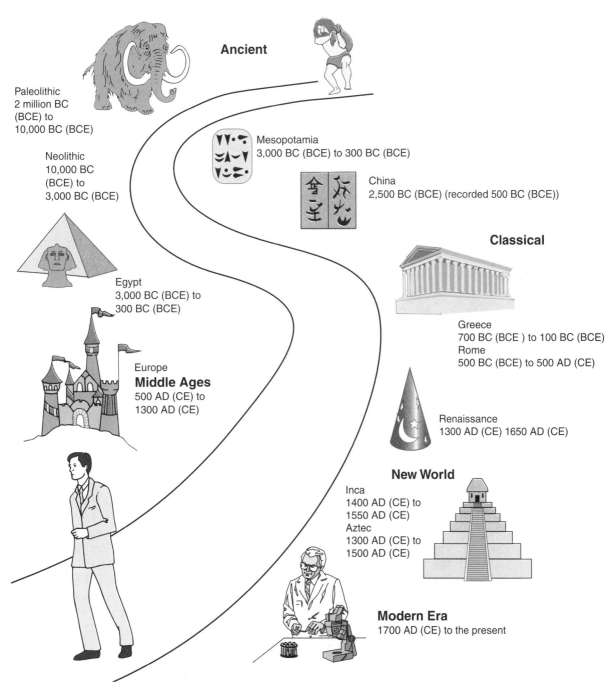

Figure 2–1 Timeline: The road to progress.

present-day Persian Gulf that the use of effective drugs was first systematically recorded.

MESOPOTAMIA (3000–300 BC [BCE])

Mesopotamia gave rise to such powerful cultures as Sumer, Assyria, and Babylon. Their writings consisted in wedge-shaped cuneiform characters impressed on clay tablets (Fig. 2–2). More than 800 of these tablets have been found, some of which recorded medical information, including herbal recipes and magic charms to exorcise the evil spirits that the Mesopotamians believed caused illness. Over 500 remedies from plant, mineral, and other sources have been deciphered. Ingredients included wine, beer, honey, oil, and aqueous extracts; and the processes used to make these medicines included filtering and boiling. Babylon's most famous king, Hammurabi (1792–1750 BC), compiled a system of laws called the *Code of Hammurabi*. These laws, which included a section of ethical standards for Babylonian healers, was drawn from even earlier Sumerian laws and customs. Its basis was "an eye for an eye," and it included patient compensation for any harm done by a practitioner.

EGYPT (3000–300 BC [BCE])

The Egyptian civilization sprang up along the banks of the Nile River concurrently with the cultures of Mesopotamia. Egyptian priests of Per-Ankh (House of Life) practiced religion and medicine together, and their temples also served as areas of healing (ancient hospitals?). One famous priest-physician was Imhotep of the Third Dynasty (c. 2620 BC). Upon his death, he was deified. Later, he was honored by the Greeks as well, who associated him with the Greek god of healing, Aesclepius. The ancient Egyptian god of learning—and patron deity of physicians—was Thoth. Egyptian priest-physicians would appeal to Thoth as they used their medicines, which included antacids, opium, alkaline laxatives, belladonna, sedatives, diuretics, and astringents. They utilized exotic herbs and strange ingredients in their prescriptions; however, all medicine was carefully dispensed to patients according to explicit directions compiled in medical papyri. These directions included exact dosages and descriptions of the manner in which the medicines were to be taken, as well as the appropriate magical spells and incantations. One of the longest of these medical papyri, called the Ebers Papyrus, has a full section devoted to pharmacology. This papyrus, which dates from the Eighteenth Dynasty (1525–1504 BC), was discovered in the mid-1800s by Georg Ebers. It contains more than 900 diagnoses and prescriptions, measures 65 feet, and includes 108 separate pages.

CHINA (FROM 2500 BC [BCE])

The early history of Chinese medicine and pharmacy is lost in legend because much of this knowledge was transmitted orally. The earliest known texts con-

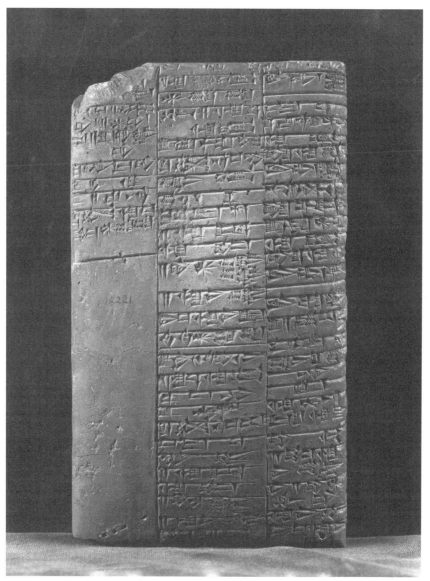

Figure 2–2 Cuneiform medical tablet from Nippur, a city of ancient Mesopotamia. [Photograph courtesy of the University of Pennsylvania Museum, Philadelphia.]

cerning drugs date from the last five centuries BC. These texts were inscriptions on wooden and bamboo slats. They gave drug quantities, dosage forms, and doses, together with symptoms for indicated drugs. In 1596 AD (CE), a compilation of drugs from more than 1000 plant and nearly 450 animal sources was written. Another work, called the Pen-ts'ao Kang-mu, by China's naturalist Li Shih-chen contained more than 11,000 prescriptions. It represented 30 years of work and travel through the country. The Chinese believed there was a remedy for every illness, and that almost everything could have a medicinal use. This belief was tied to the philosophical ides of the balance of living forces. They also believed the drugs displayed characteristics similar to the conditions they helped to cure; thus, they sought red ingredients for cardiovascular ailments and yellow for liver and bile ailments. Chinese drugs include gingsing (an herbal medicine), ephedra (from which we get ephedrine, a bronchodilator), cassia bark (possibly used as an antiemetic), rhubarb (a laxative), and camphor (a medicine to counteract itching).

Classical Era (700 BC [BCE]–500 AD [CE])

By the time of the ancient Greeks and Romans, medicine and surgery became grounded upon physical experience supplemented by religious beliefs and ritual practices. There were doctors and salaried public medical officers in Athens, as well as private pharmacies and written pharmacopoeias.

GREECE (700–100 BC [BCE])

Classical Greek civilization produced great philosophical and scientific advances, many in the area of medicine. One such natural philosopher was Hippocrates, known today as the Father of Medicine and author of the Hippocratic Oath (Insight 2–1), a code for ethical conduct and practice by doctors. Born in 460 BC on the Island of Cos, a teaching and healing center of that time, Hippocrates dismissed the efficacy of superstitious beliefs and magical incantations in healing arts, stressing careful clinical observation instead. Hippocrates cited over 400 drugs in his writings. Later, after the Greek and Mesopotamian world was conquered by the Macedonian Alexander the Great (323 BC), Greek civilization combined with Near-Eastern culture to produce the Hellenistic civilization, which also spread to Egypt. Another famous Greek physician was Dioscorides, who lived in the first century. He compiled a formulary of medicines arranged according to drug source—as plant, animal, or mineral. He described more than 700 plants, trees, wines, and spices. Some types of drugs used in Greece were opium, emetics, expectorants, diuretics, hyoscyamus, (which contains atropine), and squill (which is similar to digitalis).

ROME (500 BC [BCE]–500 AD [CE])

By the end of the first century BC, Rome had conquered the Hellenistic world, and Greek medical knowledge passed to Rome. The Greek-born physician Galen (131–200 AD) was the most famous physician of his time and for centuries to come. His books on every aspect of medicine were used in the first European universities of the thirteenth century. He practiced and taught medicine and pharmacy in Rome. Galen's teachings described health as the perfect balance of four

INSIGHT 2–1 | THE HIPPOCRATIC OATH

I swear by Apollo the physician, by Aesculapius, Hygeia, and Panacea, and I take to witness all the gods, all the goddesses, to keep according to my ability and my judgment the following oath:

To consider dear to me as my parents him who taught me this art; to live in common with him and if necessary to share my goods with him; to look upon his children as my own brothers, to teach them this art if they so desire without fee or written promise; to impart to my sons and the sons of the master who taught me and the disciples who have enrolled themselves and have agreed to the rules of the profession, but to these alone, the precepts and the instruction. I will prescribe a regimen for the good of my patients according to my ability and my judgment and never do harm to anyone. To please no one will I prescribe a deadly drug, nor give advice which may cause his death. Nor will I give a woman a pessary to procure abortion. But I will preserve the purity of my life and my art. I will not cut for stone, even for patients in whom the disease is manifest; I will leave this operation to be performed by practitioners (specialists in this art). In every house where I come I will enter only for the good of my patients, keeping myself far from all intentional ill-doing and all seduction, and especially from the pleasures of love with women or with men, be they free or slaves. All that may come to my knowledge in the exercise of my profession or in daily commerce with men, which ought not to be spread abroad, I will keep secret and will never reveal. If I keep this oath faithfully, may I enjoy my life and practice my art, respected by all men and in all times; but if I swerve from it or violate it, may the reverse be my lot.

biles in the human body—blood, phlegm, yellow bile, and black bile. Galen described 473 drugs of vegetable, animal, or mineral origin and a large number of formulas. He was the first to make rosewater ointment (cold cream). He described remedies and drug components in his book *On the Art of Healing.* His medicines, in the form of syrups, ointments, and tinctures, were abstracted from soaking or boiling plants. Galen also carefully identified the type and age of his specimens. Another man of science of this era was Pliny the Elder. He was a Roman naturalist who compiled a *Historia Naturalis.* One of Pliny's prescriptions was gold ointment. He believed so strongly in this medicine that he prescribed it for everything from ulcers to hemorrhoids.

The Middle Ages (500–1300)

With the fall of the Western Roman Empire in the fifth century, learning and recording of knowledge were drastically curtailed in Europe. But a few of the works from the classical era survived because a religious order of monks, the Benedictines, saved them. Their monasteries served as educational and medical centers during

Europe's Dark Ages (500–1000). The monks studied and made copies of many of the earlier writings. They also grew herbs in monastery gardens. While the West seemed stagnant in the stream of learning, the East continued to make advances. The Eastern empire flourished under Constantinople, preserving the Greek and Roman culture intact and borrowing much from China. Islam, too, built on the classical foundations. The greatest physician of Islam was Ibn Sina, known in Latin as Avicenna (980–1037). His chief medical contribution was the *Canon Medicinae,* which contained in five books the medicines and medical knowledge used by Arabs, Persians, and Indians of the time. Much of his *Canon* derived from Dioscorides and Galen, with his own impressive additions. Translated into Latin, his work was the accepted authority in Europe until the seventeenth century. Arab scholars introduced drugs from the Near East, the Orient, and Africa into the *materia medica* (recorded medical knowledge). They also added new dosage forms such as syrups, juleps, and confections using sugar or honey, which confounded the Western notion that the only good medicines were bitter or bad-tasting.

The Renaissance (1300–1650)

After the first Crusades, Europe began a new age of enlightenment known as the Renaissance. Spurred by new contact with the East (where classical culture never died), Europeans rediscovered classical art, literature, science, and medicine. From this era came Leonardo da Vinci's studies of anatomic detail, which were of great interest to medicine. Also at this time Dioscorides' *De Materia Medica* was made available in many editions in Europe.

Another figure from this era was a man who studied at many universities, but obtained no medical degree. Nevertheless, his ideas would greatly advance pharmacology. Known as Paracelsus (1493–1541), he traveled throughout Europe practicing medicine and searching for knowledge, both medical and alchemical (Fig. 2–3). He was appointed to a post at the University of Basel where his lectures were very controversial because he found fault with much of the works of Galen, Hippocrates, and Avicenna. Paracelsus claimed that illness was the result of "seeds of disease" which attacked some body organs. He understood the chemical nature of the body and maintained that illnesses could be cured by using chemically prepared medicines. His understanding of metallurgy and natural chemistry was the key to his discoveries (see Insight 2–2). These discoveries included using precisely measured doses of mercury compounds to treat syphilis. He also discovered laudanum (an opium derivative), combined sulfuric acid and alcohol to produce an ether-type drug, and added sulfur, mercury, lead, iron, arsenic, copper sulfate, and potassium sulfate to the known *materia medica.* In addition, Paracelsus described the circulation as the "sap of life" and treated epilepsy as a disease, not as a demonic possession. Although Paracelsus was denounced by the medical establishment, he effected many cures after orthodox medical practice had failed.

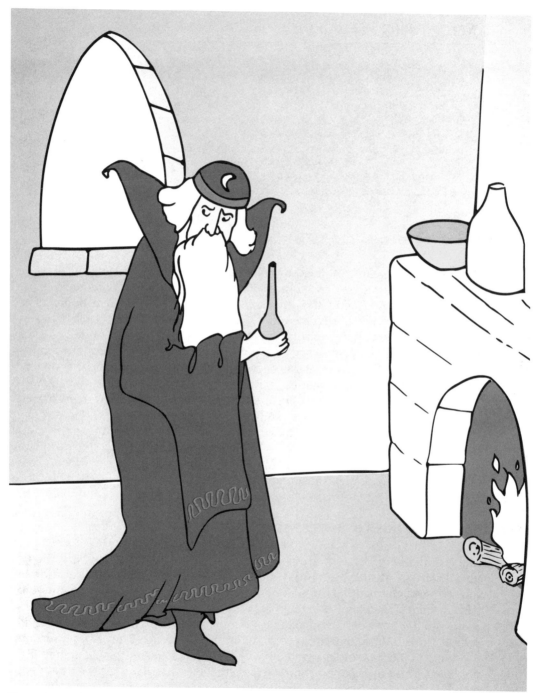

Figure 2–3 The alchemist.

INSIGHT 2–2 | ALCHEMY

Though believed to have begun in Egypt long before the birth of Christ, alchemy gained prominence during the Renaissance through men like Paracelsus. Alchemy was the art practiced by those who searched for the grand *arcanum*—the secret of turning base metals into gold. A later goal of the alchemist was to restore balance (health) through the use of chemical remedies. These men searched for the philosopher's stone—a magical substance that could endow its owner with great powers, including invisibility. They also looked for the magical elixir of life. While experimenting, cataloguing, and recording their findings, alchemists established the foundations for such modern-day sciences as pharmacology and chemistry.

New World Era (recorded c. 1500)

Before the European conquest, Brazilian Indians used the powdered roots of ipecacuanha (ipecac) to treat a form of amebic diarrhea. Pre-Columbian Mexicans used tobacco (nicotiana) and hallucinogenics (sacred mushrooms). The Incas, natives of the Peruvian Andes, used two medicines still used today: cocaine and quinine (used to treat malaria). They found that the chewed leaves of the coca shrub could be used as a poultice for wounds, so that the wounds became numb. Coca leaves were also given to the long-distance message runners who provided the communication system for the Andes kingdoms. When swallowed, the leaves acted as a euphoric and stimulant. Coca leaves were also used in the Inca religious ceremonies. To keep up with its demand, the Incas maintained coca plantations using slave labor. Another civilization of the New World—the Aztecs found in Mexico—also used herbs, plants, and seeds as medicines. A Spanish physician named Martin de la Cruz compiled a work on Aztec medicines; this work was translated into Latin in 1552 and taken to Europe.

Modern Era (late 1700s to the present)

Much of the knowledge of drugs from early civilizations has been lost. Some ancient drugs are still used today, but these represent only a small portion of modern medicine. During the eighteenth century, pharmacy and medicine went through many changes. Though great advances were made, there were no laws to govern this science. One result was that many useless compounds were still popular forms of treatment. Toward the latter half of the 1700s, two important advances in pharmacology occurred. In 1785, William Withering of England discovered the use of digitalis, obtained from the foxglove plant, for the treatment of heart disease. Then, in 1796, another English physician, Edward Jenner, introduced an immunization for smallpox, which had been one of Europe's great killers.

In the nineteenth century, pharmaceutical chemistry began to emerge as an individual science. A subdivision of this science was pharmacology. Attention was given to dosage accuracy, and standards for drug preparation were established. Another great advance was made in 1815 when Frederick Serturner, a German pharmacist, isolated the alkaloid morphine from opium. Other drugs discovered (and rediscovered) were quinine, strychnine (a poisonous alkaloid), atropine, and codeine.

More pharmacologic progress has probably been made in the past fifty years than in all the previous centuries combined. This makes the twentieth century one of fantastic progress. It is estimated that almost 80% of the drugs currently utilized were not available even thirty years ago. In this era, laws were developed to protect the population from harmful or hazardous drugs. Some of the major breakthroughs in pharmacology during the twentieth century include Paul Ehrlich's introduction of salvarson for the treatment of syphilis in 1907 and his introduction of the concept of chemotherapy; Frederick Banting and Charles Best's discovery of insulin for the treatment of diabetes mellitus in 1922; Alexander Fleming's discovery of penicillin in 1929; and Jonas Salk's discovery of a vaccine for poliomyelitis in 1955. Synthetic chemicals are now being developed at dizzying speed. Drugs and drug categories are also being discovered. These include the immunomodulators—drugs used to treat autoimmune diseases and fight against the body's rejection of transplants—and protease inhibitors, which fight AIDS.

Table 2–1 provides a summary of the history of pharmacology, as recounted here.

Table 2–1 History of Pharmacology

Prehistoric Era		Plants, herbs, magic
		Drawings of plants on bones
Ancient Era		
Mesopotamia		Cuneiform writing, magic
	Hammurabi	Code of Hammurabi
Egypt	Imhotep	Priest-religion-medicine
	Thoth	God of medicine
	Ebers Papyrus	Medical papyri
China		Writings on wood and bamboo
	Li Shih-chen	Pen-ta'ao Kang-mu
Classical Era		
Greece	Hippocrates	Father of Medicine
	Dioscorides	Medicinal formulary
Rome	Galen	*On the Art of Healing*
	Pliny the Elder	*Historia Naturalis*
Middle Ages		
Europe	Benedictine monks	Preserved knowledge
The East	Avicenna	*Canon Medicinae*
		(cont.)

Table 2–1   (cont.)

The Renaissance		
Europe	Leonardo da Vinci	Anatomic detail
	Paracelsus	Alchemy
New World Era		
Peru	Inca	Coca leaves
Brazil	Natives	Ipecac
Mexico	Aztecs, natives	Tobacco, mushrooms
Modern Era		
England	Withering	Digitalis
	Jenner	Smallpox vaccine
Germany	Serturner	Isolated morphine
20th CentZury		
	Ehrlich	Salvarson, chemotherapy
	Banting and Best	Insulin
	Fleming	Penicillin
	Salk	Polio vaccine

Drug Sources

Drugs in use today come from five main sources: plants, animals, minerals, the chemical laboratory, and the genetic engineering laboratory.

At one time, plants were nearly the only source of medicines available. Today, however, only a few drugs are still derived directly from plant sources (Fig. 2–4). Examples of current drugs made from plants include atropine from the roots of the belladonna plant (deadly nightshade), digitalis from the leaves of the purple foxglove, and morphine from the seeds of the opium poppy.

Animals (Fig. 2–5) provide a source for some drugs, particularly hormones. Cattle and hog endocrine glands were the best available source of hormones prior to the advent of genetic engineering. We describe drugs derived from hogs as *porcine* and those from cattle as *bovine.* Thus, thyroglobulin (Proloid)—a purified extract of hog thyroid gland—is porcine in origin, while thrombin (Thrombogen)—

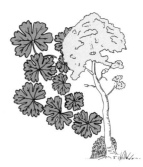

Figure 2–4   Plants are sources of some drugs in use today.

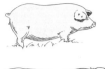
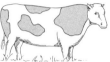

Figure 2–5   Animals are sources of some drugs in use today.

a topical hemostatic—is bovine in origin. Insulin is both bovine and porcine because it is obtained from the pancreas of cattle and hogs.

Minerals (Fig. 2–6), such as calcium, magnesium, and silver salts in several forms, are used in some pharmacologic agents. For example, Tums and Mylanta are antacids that contain calcium (Tums) and magnesium (Mylanta) hydroxides, and Silvadene creme is an antimicrobial agent that contains silver salts. Even gold is used, as in Solganal, which is an antiarthritic agent.

The fourth major source of drugs is chemical synthesis in the laboratory (Fig. 2–7). There are two ways for drugs to be *synthesized,* i.e., put together. *Synthetic drugs* are drugs that are synthesized from laboratory chemicals; *semisynthetic drugs* are drugs that start with a natural substance, then are altered by chemical processes. The vast majority of modern drugs are either synthetic or semisynthetic. Meperidine (Demerol) is an example of a synthetic drug; it is made from chemicals, but its pain-relieving effects are similar to those of opium. Many penicillins—like amoxicillin—are semisynthetic drugs. They are originally derived from a natural fungus (*Penicillium*), but they are altered by chemical means.

The newest source of drugs is the genetic engineering laboratory. **Recombinant DNA technology** (also referred to as *genetic engineering* or *biotechnology*) is a process that allows scientists to produce proteins from bacteria—proteins that were previously available only from animals. That is, molecular biologists use bacteria as tiny factories to produce the proteins they need to make drugs. They do this by altering the DNA of bacteria such as *Escherichia coli* (*E. coli*). How? By physically inserting a gene into the DNA of a single *E. coli* cell—a gene that *codes for* (tells the cell to make) a certain protein (see Fig. 2–8). Once one cell has this inserted gene in its DNA, it becomes a miniature copying machine, producing daughter cells that have daughter cells that have daughter cells . . . each with the new gene and each

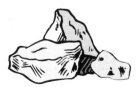

Figure 2–6   Minerals are sources of some drugs in use today.

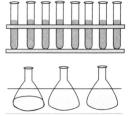

Figure 2–7 Synthetic and semisynthetic drugs are produced in a chemical laboratory.

producing the desired protein. As this reproduction process occurs very rapidly, large volumes of the desired protein can be obtained quickly.

Among the drugs produced by biotechnology are human insulin (Humulin), human growth hormone (Nutropin), and the thrombolytic agent altepase (Activase). Such genetically engineered proteins do not cause the adverse side effects—e.g., immune or allergic reactions—often seen in the long-term use of drugs from animal sources. Drugs like these are always administered by injection; they cannot be taken orally because they are proteins, which are digested when consumed.

Drug Nomenclature

The term drug nomenclature refers to the system(s) of naming drugs. Each drug has several names—usually, its chemical name, its generic name, and its trade name—and each of these names is used for a specific purpose. (See Table 2–2.)

The chemical name for a drug has meaning for chemists. This name is a precise, systematic description of the chemical composition and molecular structure of the drug.

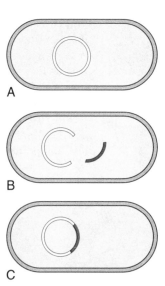

Figure 2–8 Genetic engineering: (**a**) *Escherichia coli* DNA. (**b**) Desired gene is inserted into bacterial DNA. (**c**) Bacterial DNA with recombinant gene.

Table 2–2 Generic, Chemical, and Brand Names of Three Drugs

Generic	Chemical	Brand
Bupivacaine hydrochloride	2-Piperidinecarboxamide or 1-butyl-*N*-(2,6-dimethylphenyl) monohydrochloride monohydrate	Marcaine Sensorcaine
Iohexol	*N*,*N*′-Bis(2,3-dihydroxypropyl)-5-[*N*-(2,3-dihydroxypropyl)acetamido]-2,4,6-triiodoisophthalamide	Omnipaque
Ampicillin sodium	(2*S*, 5*R*, 6*R*)-6-[(*R*)-2-Amino-2-phenylacetamido]-3,3-dimethyl-7-oxo-4-thia-1-azabicyclo[3.2.0] heptane-2-carboxylic acid	Omnipen

The generic, or nonproprietary, name for a drug is selected by its original developer and approved by the United States Adopted Name Council (USAN). The generic name does not belong to any one company, so it is not capitalized. Rather the generic name is the official name used in the *United States Pharmacopoeia and National Formulary (USP/NF)* (see Chapter 3), and is most useful when comparing similar drugs manufactured by different companies. It is important to recognize that some variations exist between generic drugs produced by different manufacturers.

☞ In this text, the generic name of a drug is listed first, followed by the trade name in parentheses, e.g., midazolam (Versed).

The trade name, also referred to as the brand name or proprietary name, is the name selected by the pharmaceutical manufacturer and used to market the drug. By law, a drug manufacturer has exclusive rights to market a new drug for seventeen years. After these exclusive rights have expired, other companies may produce equivalent drugs under different trade names. For example, a local anesthetic, bupivacaine, is sold under two brand names: Marcaine and Sensorcaine. Sometimes, trade names—like aspirin—become so popular that they are adopted as generic names.

Drug Classifications

Drug classifications group similar drugs, or drugs used for similar purposes. We can classify drugs by what they do, what they affect, and what they are; thus, common classification categories include

- *Therapeutic action:* what they do for a patient; e.g., analgesics relieve pain.
- *Physiologic action:* what they do in the body; e.g., histamine receptor antagonists block histamine reception.

- *Affected body system:* what they affect; e.g., cardiovascular agents affect the heart and circulatory system.
- *Chemical type:* what they are; e.g., barbiturates are a class of chemical compounds derived from barbituric acid.

Drugs may be cross-referenced in multiple categories. For example, ranitidine (Zantac) is categorized therapeutically as an antacid, physiologically as a histamine receptor antagonist, and by body system as a gastric agent. Each classification category has several subcategories, as shown in Table 2–3. Drugs having multiple therapeutic effects are classified in more than one subcategory. For example, aspirin relieves pain, fever, and inflammation, so it is classified as an analgesic, an antipyretic, and an anti-inflammatory agent—three different therapeutic subcategories. Therapeutic-action subcategories of drugs frequently used from the sterile back table include antibiotics, anticoagulants, anti-inflammatory agents, local anesthetics, and hemostatics.

Drugs are also classified by how they may be obtained. The distinction between prescription and nonprescription or over-the-counter (OTC) drugs is a legal classification (see Chapter 3).

Table 2–3 Drug Classification Categories and Subcategories

Therapeutic Action

Analgesic
Anticoagulant
Anti-inflammatory
Antipyretic
Sedative
Thrombolytic

Physiologic Action

alpha-Adrenergic blocker
Cholinergic
Histamine receptor antagonist
Muscle relaxant antagonist
Vasoconstrictor

Body System

Cardiovascular agent
Dermatologic agent
Ophthalmic preparation
Urinary tract agent

Chemical Type

Barbiturate
Benzodiazepine
Narcotic
Oxytocic

Medication Orders

Prescriptions

When treatment requires a specific drug, a licensed physician or designee such as a physician's assistant (PA) or nurse practitioner (NP) writes a prescription for the drug. State governments have the power to regulate which medical professionals write prescriptions, so there are variations in practice from state to state.

Figure 2–9 shows a typical prescription form. As shown, prescriptions must include the date, the name of the patient, the name of the drug, the dosage, the route of administration, and the frequency or time of administration. It must also bear the prescriber's signature. Notice that the printed form contains the name, address, telephone number, and DEA number of the prescriber. The Drug Enforcement Agency (DEA) requires that this number be listed on any prescription for a controlled substance (see Chapter 3). A written prescription usually designates the drug by trade name, but may indicate that a generic substitution is permissible. When writing prescriptions, physicians (or their

John W. Smith, M.D.

812-888-5893   Medical Building #8   Anywhere, IN 48888

For _____ *JANE DOE* _____ Age ___ 21

Address _____ *4444 End Avenue Anywhere, IN* _____ Date *2/14/99*

RX

Amoxicillin 500mg   #21

$\overline{i}$ po tid X $\overline{i}$ wk

refill _*prn*_ times

non-refill _____

label _____

_____ *John W Smyth*

dispense as written M.D.   may substitute   M.D.

DEA. NO. AS-0000000

IN License #01010101

Figure 2–9 A typical prescription form.

designees) use abbreviations and symbols (Table 2–4) for dosages, frequency, and administration routes. Pharmacists interpret these symbols and give the drugs to the patient, along with instructions for proper use. Today, many pharmacies have computer systems that provide printouts of such important drug information as side effects, precautions, normal usage, and storage.

Hospital Medication Orders

In the hospital setting, any medications to be administered to the patient must be ordered by a licensed physician or designee and written on a physician's order sheet. In surgery, the **medication order** may be one of several types:

> *Standing orders:* A standing order, or *protocol,* is used for common situations requiring a standard treatment. For example, a standing order may be in place stating that all surgical patients receive 15 milliliters of sodium citrate (Bicitra) by mouth 30 minutes before surgery.
>
> *Verbal orders:* Verbal orders are commonplace in surgery, as a surgeon may request a particular drug to be administered either from the sterile field or by the anesthesia provider.

Table 2–4 **Abbreviations for Anatomical and Administration Directions**

AD	right ear
AS	left ear
AU	bilateral ears
OD	right eye
OS	left eye
OU	bilateral eyes
os	mouth
aa	of each
ad	to, up to
ad lib	as desired
amt	amount
c̄	with
dc, DC	discontinue
et	and
KVO, TKO	keep vein open, to keep open
npo, NPO	nothing by mouth (os)
per	by means of, by
qs	quantity sufficient
Rx	take
s̄	without
ss	one half
sig	label
sos	once if necessary
stat	immediately

Stat orders: Often given verbally, stat orders indicate that a drug is to be administered immediately and one time only.

PRN orders: PRN stands for *pro re nata,* which means that the drug may be given as needed. For example, during septoplasty performed under local anesthesia, meperidine (Demerol) may be administered PRN to reduce patient discomfort.

In surgery, drugs needed during a procedure are listed on the surgeon's preference card. As shown in Figure 2–10, the preference card should list all pertinent information, such as drug strength and quantity.

Medication orders usually contain four basic parts: drug name, dosage, route of administration, and frequency. Many abbreviations are used to represent drug forms, dosages, routes, and timing of administration. Dosages are stated in a particular unit of measure, usually in the metric system, and abbreviated, such as 300 mg, 10 mL, or 1,000 units. The route of administration is usually abbreviated; for example, if a drug is to be given intravenously, it is designated as IV. The frequency or time of administration is also clearly stated and is often abbreviated; for example, if the drug is to be taken four times a day, it is designated QID. Table 2–5 lists common abbreviations used to represent frequency of drug administration.

Drug Distribution Systems

Dispensing of prescription drugs is the responsibility of a licensed pharmacist. That is, pharmacists must *release* drugs, either directly to patients or to the physician or surgeon who orders them. In hospitals, drugs are often released for storage so they can be distributed as necessary.

☞ In all medical facilities, *controlled substances* (such as morphine) must be stored in a double-locked cupboard, drawer or box once they have been released from the pharmacy. Each shift, a designated person is usually in charge of the key to the narcotics box or cupboard. At the beginning and end of each shift, two persons count the drugs to verify proper documentation of use.

Distribution systems for drugs used in surgery vary among institutions. In large hospitals, a satellite pharmacy within the surgical suite may dispense drugs as needed for each procedure. Other, often smaller, facilities may maintain a medication room or cabinet (Fig. 2–11) where they store frequently used drugs, such as antibiotics and local anesthetics. In addition, most hospitals utilize a system of mobile drug carts, which must be exchanged for restocking after the drugs are used. For example, emergency-response drug carts, known as *crash carts,* are used for cardiac arrest and other emergency situations. Such carts are often restocked on an exchange basis in order to assure the immediate availability of all necessary drugs.

REGIONAL MEDICAL CENTER
SURGEON PREFERENCE CARD AND REQUISITION

Patient name: Jane Doe
Procedure date: 01/31/99
Scheduled time: 0730
Surgeon: Meier, C.
Procedure: Cataract extraction with IOL, O.D.

Item code	Item description	Req.	Quantity Picked	Chgd
	STERILE SUPPLIES			
001957	Steridrape 1060 3M	1		
005006	Skin scrub tray	1		
000574	Glove sterile 7	1		
005890	Custom pack - eye	1		
	INSTRUMENTS			
002040	Capsule polisher	1		
001993	Irrigating cystitome	1		
011005	Phaco tubing	1		
009505	Cataract set - Meier	1		
011013	Phaco handpiece	1		
	MEDICATIONS			
002365	BSS 15 mL	2		
012032	Bio-Cor Shield	1		
002367	BSS Plus 500 mL	1		
218965	Dexamethasone 4 mg	1		
218966	Celestone 3 mg	1		
	Hold if uses shield			
012164	Ancef 50 mg	1		
	Hold if uses shield			
444364	Carbastat 1 amp	1		
417665	Maxitrol ointment	1		
010433	Opthetic gtts	1		
359003	Lidocaine 2% 50mL w/ epi 1:200,000	1		
359004	Bupivicaine 0.5%	1		
010492	Epinephrine 1:1000 1cc	1		
437283	Wydase 150 units	1		
455849	Healon .85 mL	1		
455850	Healon .4 mL	1		
	Hold			
238934	Tobradex gtts	1		
567392	Vancomycin 10 mg	1		

SURGEON SPECIAL REQUESTS

*Add 0.3 cc epinephrine, 2 mg dexamethasone, and 10 mg of Vancomycin to 500 cc bottle of BSS plus.

*Add remaining dexamethasone (2mg) to celestone for injection at end of case. (Hold if using shield)

*Mix 1 gm Ancef with 10 cc NaCl– give 0.5 cc of solution for injection at end of case (hold if using shield).

*Do not add Wydase to anesthetic agent until just prior to use.

*Combine 2% lidocaine w/ epi (5cc), bupivicaine 0.5% (5cc), and Wydase 150 units for injection.

Figure 2–10 A computerized surgeon's preference card lists medications required for the procedure.

Table 2–5 **Abbreviations for Frequency of Medication Administration**

bid	twice a day
h, hr	hour
prn, PRN	as necessary
	(*pro re nata*)
q	every
qh	every hour
q2h	every 2 hours
qid	four times a day
tid	three times a day
stat	immediately

Drugs Forms or Preparations

Drugs come in many different forms or preparations. Drugs may be in solid, semi-solid, liquid, or gaseous form (Fig. 2–12). The form of drug administered affects both the onset of drug actions and the intensity of the body's response to the drug. Liquids, for instance, tend to act more quickly than solids; and gases or vapors tend to be even faster. Drug form also dictates route of administration. For example, the antibiotic Neosporin comes in ointment (semisolid) form, which must be applied topically only. Some drugs are available in more than one form. For example, lidocaine (Xylocaine) is available in jelly for topical application and

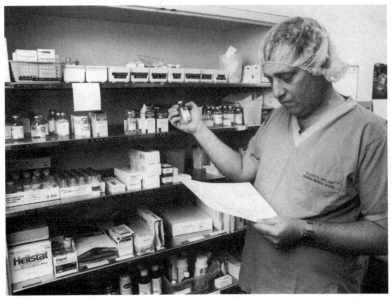

Figure 2–11 A medication cabinet in surgery.

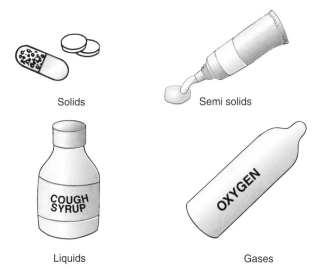

Solids   Semi solids

Liquids   Gases

Figure 2–12 Drugs are available in several forms or preparations.

in solutions of various strengths for injection. Drug forms are often abbreviated in drug orders. Table 2–6 lists several common abbreviations.

SOLIDS

Many drugs come prepared in solid form. These drugs may be in capsule (cap) or tablet (tab) form and are administered orally. Capsules are gelatin cases containing a drug in powder or granule form; tablets are a compressed form of the drug, usually combined with inert ingredients. Capsules and tablets are rarely used in surgery because oral administration is required. In most cases surgical patients must be kept NPO (nothing by mouth), or they may be under a general anesthesia and unable swallow.

Some drugs come in powder form in glass vials. Such powders must be mixed with a liquid (reconstituted) to form a solution so they can be administered by injection. For example, several antibiotics administered in surgery are powders that must be reconstituted with sterile water or a sodium chloride solution (saline) to make an injectable solution. Other drugs, such as dantrolene

Table 2–6 **Abbreviations for Drug Forms or Preparations**

cap	capsule
gtts	drops
soln	solution
susp	suspension
tab	tablet
ung	ointment

(Dantrium)—an infrequently used, yet important skeletal muscle relaxant—also come in powder form and must be reconstituted prior to use.

SEMISOLIDS

Semisolid preparations include creams, foams, gels, ointments, and suppositories. Examples of semisolid drugs used in surgery include lidocaine (Xylocaine) jelly for topical anesthesia, Silvadene creme for burns, and Neosporin ointment for wound dressing.

LIQUIDS

Several types of liquid drug preparations are available. They may be **solution**, in which drugs are fully dissolved in liquid medium (e.g., water, alcohol, or saline). Many solutions are used in surgery, including intravenous solutions of dextrose, antibiotic irrigation solutions, and heparin irrigation solution.

Drugs in liquid form may also be administered orally, as *elixirs* (sweetened solutions of alcohol) or *syrups* (sweetened aqueous solutions). But elixirs and syrups are rarely, if ever, used in surgery. Drugs may also be in **suspension** form where solid particles float in (are suspended) in a liquid. Suspensions must be shaken prior to administration to evenly distribute particles throughout the liquid. Suspensions used in surgery include Cortisporin otic, used in ear surgery, and Celestone, an anti-inflammatory used in ophthalmology.

GASES

The only common medications available in gas form are inhalation anesthetic agents. These include nitrous oxide and volatile liquids such as halothane (see Chapter 13).

Drug Administration Routes

Drugs are formulated to be administered by a specific route. In addition to drug form, the route by which a drug is given can affect onset time and body response. Drugs may be administered by many different routes, only a few of which are used commonly in surgery. All drug orders state route of administration, usually in abbreviated form (Table 2–7).

The oral route (PO) is the simplest and most common way to administer many drugs. Drugs may be ingested (swallowed) or allowed to dissolve, either in the cheek (buccally) or under the tongue (sublingually). Most drugs are readily absorbed through the mucosa of the gastrointestinal tract. Certain drugs may irritate the gastrointestinal mucosa and should therefore be given with food. Other drugs may be inactivated by increased amounts of digestive enzymes and so are best taken between meals. When drugs are administered orally, onset of action is

Table 2–7 **Abbreviations for Drug Administration Routes**

IM	intramuscular
IV	intravenous
PO, po	per os, orally
SC, subq	subcutaneously

usually slower and duration of effect is usually longer than with other routes. Some drugs, however, are completely inactivated by the digestive process and therefore must not be given orally. Insulin, a hormone, and heparin, an anticoagulant, are not effective when administered orally. Although few drugs are given by mouth in surgery, one exception is oral administration of sodium citrate (Bicitra), which is given preoperatively to neutralize gastric acid (Chapter 12).

Many drugs are administered topically for **local effect.** Creams and ointments may be spread onto skin; for example, an antibiotic ointment may be applied directly on a surgical wound. Other drugs may be instilled into a mucous membrane–lined area, such as the eye, nose, urethra, vagina, or rectum. Mucous membranes generally have excellent blood supply, so absorption is usually quite rapid. For example, lidocaine (Xylocaine) jelly may be instilled into the urethra as topical anesthesia for cystoscopy. Topical antibiotic irrigation is common in surgery, in which case an antibiotic solution is poured or squirted into the surgical site. Inhalation is another topical route for drug administration. Some asthmatic drugs are administered through a nebulizer—a device that converts liquid drugs into an inhalable mist. The drug is absorbed in the bronchi of the lungs, providing local relief of bronchoconstriction. Anesthetic gases and vapors are also administered via inhalation, but these drugs exert **systemic** rather than local effects.

The majority of drugs used in surgery are administered **parenterally**, i.e., by any route OTHER than the alimentary canal (the *enteral* route). There are many parenteral routes, the most common of which are the subcutaneous, intramuscular, and intravenous routes.

Subcutaneous (SC) injections are given beneath the skin into the subcutaneous tissue layer. Common sites for subcutaneous injections are the upper lateral aspect of the arm, the anterior thigh, and the abdomen. Depending on blood supply, absorption from subcutaneous tissue is fairly rapid. Only a few drugs are administered subcutaneously in surgery; for example, heparin may be injected subcutaneously preoperatively in some cases to help prevent pulmonary embolism.

A few drugs used in surgery are administered *intramuscularly* (IM). Intramuscular injections are usually given into a large muscle mass, such as the deltoid, gluteal, or vastus lateralis. Intramuscular absorption is usually rapid due to the large absorbing surface and good blood supply. An example of a drug given IM in surgery is ketorolac (Toradol), a nonsteroidal anti-inflammatory drug (NSAID) used for postoperative pain relief.

Most drugs administered parenterally in surgery are given *intravenously* (IV), i.e., within a vein, as shown in Figure 2–13. A small catheter is inserted into

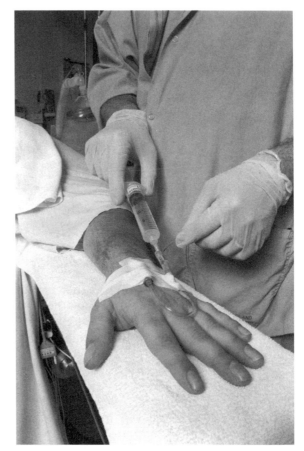

Figure 2–13 A drug may be administered by intravenous injection.

a vein, then connected to tubing called an infusion set. The infusion set is attached to a bag of intravenous fluid for administration. Drugs may then be injected as needed into sites along the tubing. Drugs may be given all at once, as a bolus, or by slow infusion. Absorption is immediate because drugs administered intravenously go directly into the bloodstream.

Other parenteral routes are used less frequently. *Intradermal* injections are given between layers of skin, as seen in tuberculin skin testing and allergy testing. A local anesthetic may be injected intradermally prior to placing an intravenous catheter, thereby reducing discomfort at the insertion site. *Intra-articular* injections (into the joint space) of anti-inflammatory agents or local anesthetics may be given after arthroscopy. *Intrathecal* injections of anesthetics or contrast media are administered into the spinal subarachnoid space. During a cardiac arrest resuscitation, a drug such as epinephrine may be injected directly into the heart; this is called an *intracardiac* injection.

Pharmacokinetics

The human body responds to drugs in varying degrees and at various rates. A body's response to a drug largely depends both upon the amount of drug given and the amount of drug actually reaching the site of action. Four basic processes—absorption, distribution, metabolism, and excretion—affect physiologic response to drugs. The study of these four processes is called **pharmacokinetics** (Table 2–8).

Absorption

For a drug to be effective, it must first be absorbed into the body. A drug is absorbed from the site of administration into the bloodstream, then carried into the systemic circulation. Speed of absorption varies by administration route and by blood supply to the area. Solubility of the drug also affects absorption. If a drug is in solid form, it must dissolve before absorption. Drugs in suspensions absorb faster than solid drugs, and solutions absorb faster than suspensions.

Oral absorption varies, depending on the drug's chemical structure as well as the pH (acidity) and motility of the gastrointestinal tract. If the digestive tract is highly motile, as seen in patients with diarrhea, ingested drugs may not be adequately absorbed. Conversely, if the patient is constipated, drugs may be fully absorbed, sometimes to toxic levels. Intramuscular absorption is rapid if water-based drug solutions are injected, and slower if the solution is oil-based. The amount and vascularization of muscle mass also affects the rate of absorption. Intravenous absorption is immediate because drugs are injected directly into the bloodstream. The absorption rate of drugs given subcutaneously is dependent upon blood supply to the area of injection.

☞ Rapid drug absorption can be undesirable in surgery when local anesthetics are used. The anesthetic agent must stay in the desired area instead of being carried away by the blood. Thus, a *vasoconstrictor,* usually epinephrine, may be added to the anesthetic agent to narrow the blood vessels and delay absorption.

Table 2–8 The Four Processes of Pharmacokinetics

Process	Body System
Absorption	Body system varies by administration route, e.g., integumentary, gastrointestinal, respiratory
Distribution	Circulatory system
Metabolism	Liver
Excretion	Kidney

Absorption of drugs given by inhalation, especially inhalation anesthetics, is rapid due to the huge numbers of capillaries in the alveoli of the lungs. Some drugs administered by inhalation (such as steroids for asthma) are specifically formulated for local effect, and so do not absorb rapidly. Mucosal tissues provide excellent absorption for some drugs due to the number of capillaries just under the mucosal surface. Common mucosal administration sites include the respiratory tract, oral cavity, and the conjunctiva. In surgery, several drugs are administered topically to mucous membranes; for example, in nasal septoplasty, cocaine-soaked packing strips may be placed directly on nasal mucosa for anesthesia.

Although most drugs are not absorbed easily through skin, some are specifically formulated to overcome the skin barrier. Such drugs are administered transdermally from patches. Scopolamine patches, for instance, are used to treat motion sickness; they release the drug slowly so it may be absorbed through skin over a period of hours.

Distribution

Once a drug has been absorbed into the bloodstream, it is transported throughout the body by systemic circulation. Drug molecules eventually diffuse out of the bloodstream to the site of action. Because drugs are carried to all parts of the body, their effects can be seen in locations other than the intended area. The amount of drug reaching the site of action depends on effective blood flow to that area and on the extent of plasma protein binding.

PLASMA PROTEIN BINDING

Not all drug molecules in the bloodstream are available to bind at the site of action. Some drug molecules bind to proteins contained in plasma—the liquid portion of blood—via a process known as **plasma protein binding.** Both the amount of plasma protein in the blood and the binding characteristics of the drug determine the extent to which a drug is bound. Some drugs are highly bound (up to 99%), some are only minimally bound, while others are not bound at all. Drugs may also compete with other drugs for binding sites, changing the amount of available drug significantly. Potential hazards arise if patients are taking different drugs that compete for the same binding sites. For instance, if a patient taking warfarin sodium (Coumadin), a highly bound anticoagulant, takes aspirin, the aspirin will bind with the same plasma protein sites, making more warfarin available than is needed (Fig. 2–14). If more than the expected amount of warfarin is available, overmedication and excessive anticoagulation may occur. Plasma protein binding is reversible. When the concentration of unbound drug in blood is lowered, either by metabolism or excretion, bound molecules are released from binding sites. The extent of plasma protein binding can prolong a drug's effects and contribute to drug–drug interactions.

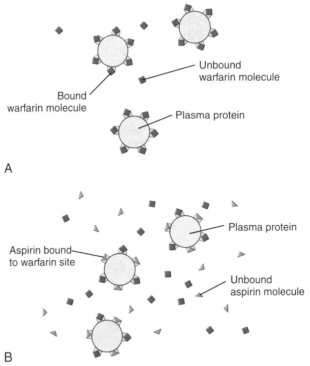

Figure 2–14 Plasma protein binding of aspirin and warfarin. (**A**) Warfarin binds to specific receptor sites on plasma proteins. (**B**) Aspirin binds to the same receptor sites, making more warfarin available.

Metabolism

The circulatory system also distributes drugs through the liver. In the liver, drugs are chemically altered via a process called *metabolism* or *biotransformation.* Liver cells (hepatocytes) contain enzymes that break down some drug molecules into other molecules called metabolites. Metabolites are usually less toxic and more easily excreted than the original drug. The effectiveness of liver enzymes depends on several factors, including patient age, concurrent drug therapy, organ disease (e.g., cirrhosis), and nutritional status. Only unbound drug molecules can be metabolized. While some drugs are completely metabolized and some are not metabolized at all, most drugs are at least partially metabolized. Some drugs are really *prodrugs;* this means they are administered in an inactive form, which is metabolized into an active drug to produce the needed effect.

All drugs taken orally enter the liver through portal circulation (Fig. 2–15) prior to entering systemic circulation. Many drugs undergo a first-pass effect, which means they may be altered or nearly inactivated when passing through the liver, potentially reducing the drug's effectiveness. Once liver enzymes begin to metabolize drug molecules, however, the enzymes are less able to metabolize additional drug; thus, repeated dosing may be necessary to overcome the first-pass effect.

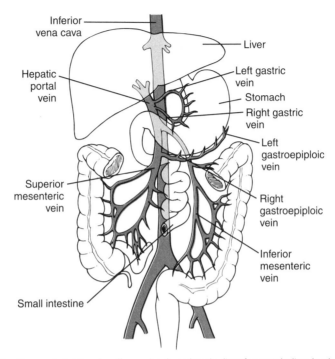

Figure 2–15 Drugs administered orally are distributed to the liver for metabolism by the hepatic portal circulation.

Labels in figure:
- Inferior vena cava
- Liver
- Hepatic portal vein
- Left gastric vein
- Stomach
- Right gastric vein
- Left gastroepiploic vein
- Superior mesenteric vein
- Right gastroepiploic vein
- Inferior mesenteric vein
- Small intestine

Excretion

Most unchanged drugs and metabolites are excreted by the kidneys and eliminated in urine (Fig. 2–16). Two renal processes remove drugs from the body: glomerular filtration and tubular secretion. Only drug molecules not bound to plasma proteins will be filtered out of blood reaching the glomerulus. How much unbound drug is filtered out depends on the glomerular filtration rate (GFR), which is dependent on blood pressure and blood flow to the kidneys. Tubular secretion uses cellular energy to force drugs and their metabolites from the bloodstream for elimination. Some drugs, depending on their characteristics and the pH of urine, may be reabsorbed and returned to circulation by tubular reabsorption.

Pharmacodynamics

Pharmacodynamics is the study of how drugs exert their effects. Several terms are used to clarify the timing of expected drug effects. The time between administration of a drug and the first appearance of effects is called the onset. The time

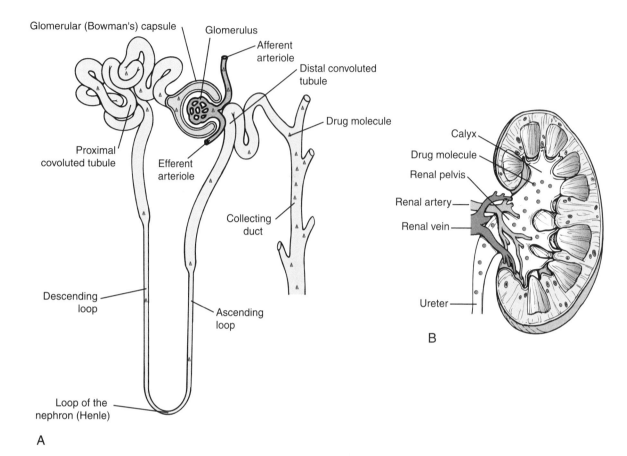

Glomerular (Bowman's) capsule

Glomerulus

Afferent arteriole

Distal convoluted tubule

Drug molecule

Proximal covoluted tubule

Efferent arteriole

Collecting duct

Descending loop

Ascending loop

Loop of the nephron (Henle)

A

Calyx

Drug molecule

Renal pelvis

Renal artery

Renal vein

Ureter

B

Figure 2–16   Most drugs are excreted by the kidney. (**A**) Drugs are removed in the nephron and (**B**) eliminated by the kidney.

between administration and maximum effect is called time to peak effect. And the time between onset and disappearance of drug effects is called the duration. Some specific mechanisms of drug actions are known, but much remains to be discovered regarding many physiologic interactions involved in drug therapy. Drugs must be able to reach the site of action and interact with cells in order to produce therapeutic effects. In most cases, drugs bind to specialized proteins, or receptors, on cell membranes. **Agonists** are drugs or chemicals that bind to a receptor, then alter some biologic function to produce an effect (Fig. 2–17). Natural agonists include neurotransmitters, such as acetylcholine (Fig. 2–17a), and hormones. Some drugs such as succinylcholine act as chemical agonists (Fig. 2–17b). **Antagonists** bind to receptor site proteins, then inhibit a response by preventing the agonist from binding (Fig. 2–17c). Antagonists are also called receptor blockers. Drug antagonism is responsible for many drug interactions,

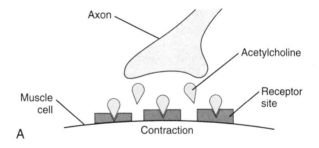

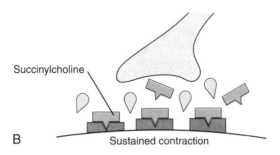

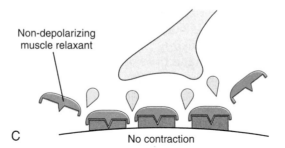

Figure 2–17 Receptor site agonist and antagonist action:
(**A**) Acetylcholine is a natural agonist.
(**B**) Succinylcholine is a chemical agonist.
(**C**) Nondepolarizing muscle relaxants act as antagonists.

some of which are not desired. Many patients are on multiple drug therapy, so potential exists for several drug–drug interactions. Multiple drugs may cancel each other out or reduce each other's effects. A drug that enhances the effect of another drug is called a *synergist*. Some drug–drug interactions may cause a dramatic increase in the intended effect of the primary drug.

Not all drug actions are receptor-type interactions. For example, mannitol—an osmotic diuretic—increases the osmotic pressure of urine; this means it reduces reabsorption of water and produces large amounts of dilute urine. Skin disinfectants such as alcohol denature the proteins in bacterial cell walls. The anticoagulant heparin neutralizes the electric charge on a plasma protein that is needed to initiate blood clotting. Antacids such as sodium bicarbonate chemically neutralize acid in the stomach.

Drug Reactions

A **side effect** is an expected but unintended effect of a drug. Side effects are rarely serious, but usually unavoidable. An example of a side effect is the drowsiness that often occurs when antihistamines are used.

Adverse effects are undesired, potentially harmful side effects of drugs. Adverse effects include drug toxicity, hypersensitivity, and idiosyncratic (unusual) reactions. Drug toxicity may be the result of accidental overdosing or failure of the body to process the drug properly, as seen in patients with kidney or liver dysfunction. In cases of drug toxicity, the primary effect of the drug may be exaggerated, such as excessive anticoagulation when taking coumarins. Some drugs may be particularly toxic to a specific organ, such as the liver, kidney, or even the ear. For example, some antibiotics are known to be ototoxic in high doses; i.e., they have the potential to damage the hearing mechanism.

Drug hypersensitivity is an adverse effect resulting from previous exposure to the drug or a similar drug. A patient may become sensitized to a drug after one or more doses, then exhibit an allergic response upon subsequent administration of the drug. An allergic response may be immediate, with symptoms ranging from mild to severe. Mild allergy symptoms include the appearance of raised patches on the skin (wheals) with itching, commonly known as hives. A severe allergic reaction, called anaphylaxis, can result in swollen bronchial passages and possible circulatory collapse (Chapter 15). Delayed allergic reactions can occur days or weeks after a drug is taken and can include fever and joint swelling.

Idiosyncratic drug effects are rare and unpredictable adverse reactions to drugs. Most idiosyncratic drug reactions are thought to occur in persons with some genetic abnormality, causing either an excessive or an inadequate response to a drug. For example, malignant hyperthermia (Chapter 15) is a life-threatening response to certain drugs, attributable to a genetic defect.

Summary

Drugs have been used throughout history to treat many conditions. The earliest sources of drugs were plants. As the healing arts developed, other sources of drugs were discovered, including animals and minerals. Today we use drugs derived from plants, animals, and minerals, as well as drugs developed in the chemistry and molecular biology laboratory.

Drugs are classified by different names and prescribing categories. The surgical technologist should be familiar with both generic and trade names of drugs used frequently in surgery. Medication orders may be in various forms in surgery, and must be interpreted precisely. The surgical technologist should also be able to utilize different drug distribution systems, depending on the system in use at the clinical facility.

Drugs come in many forms or preparations, and surgical technologists must be able to recognize the type needed for the intended purpose. While surgical technologists do not routinely administer drugs, they must still be aware of the different routes used for specific drugs. By far, the intravenous route is the most common used in surgery.

Surgical technologists should be aware of the basic physiology involved in drug therapy. Pharmacokinetics is the study of the four basic steps the body uses to process drugs: absorption, distribution, metabolism, and excretion. The study of how drugs exert their effects is called pharmacodynamics. Most drugs interact with receptors on target cell membranes to produce the desired effect. Many drugs cause expected side effects that are rarely serious. Adverse effects are undesired and potentially serious drug side effects. Knowledge of basic principles of pharmacology will provide the surgical technologist with a solid foundation on which to build an understanding of the many drugs used in surgery.

REVIEW

1. What are the sources of drugs used today? State examples.

2. How are generic drug names different from trade names?

3. How are drug classification categories helpful?

4. What types of drug orders are used in surgery?

5. Describe the drug distribution system used in your clinical facility.

6. Which drug forms/preparations and administration routes have you seen used in surgery?

7. How does the body process drugs?

8. What is a side effect? An adverse effect? Give an example of each.

CHAPTER 3

Drug Regulation

Drug Regulation
Federal Laws
State Practice Acts
Local Policies

Drug Development
Phases of Drug Testing
Marketing

Drug References
Physician's Desk Reference
United States Pharmacopoeia
   and National Formulary
Hospital Pharmacist
Data Bases

OBJECTIVES

Upon completion of this chapter you should be able to:

1 Discuss federal and state roles in regulating drugs.
2 Characterize the phases of human drug testing.
3 Obtain drug information from pharmacology resources.

KEY TERMS

Contraindication *Counter* (opposite) indication—a reason or condition that renders a particular line of treatment improper or undesirable.

Controlled substances Drugs whose dispensation is regulated by federal law because of their dependency or abuse potential.

DEA Drug Enforcement Agency; the federal agency responsible for enforcing the Controlled Substances Act.

FDA Food and Drug Administration; a division of the federal Department of Health and Human Services; responsible for monitoring drug development, manufacturing, and marketing.

Indication Condition or reason to prescribe medication or perform a procedure.

Narcotics Drugs that produce insensibility or stupor.

OTC Over-the-counter drugs; drugs that may be sold without a prescription.

PDR *Physician's Desk Reference;* a compilation of drug information obtained from pharmaceutical companies.

Prescription drugs Drugs requiring a physician's order to dispense.

USP/NF *United States Pharmacopoeia and National Formulary;* the official listing of drug information recognized by the U.S. government.

As a surgical technologist, you should be aware of federal, state, and local roles in regulating drugs and their administration. In this chapter, then, we'll present a broad overview of federal drug legislation as well as a general discussion of state and local regulation. Because new drugs are approved for use regularly, we'll also briefly consider the process that leads to this approval—drug testing and study. Finally, we'll look at available drug references, which will help you obtain information useful to your practice as a surgical technologist.

Drug Regulation

Before the twentieth century, drugs of all kinds were sold freely in the United States, both to physicians and consumers. Thus, neither physician nor consumer had any real proof of the drug's safety or effectiveness. There was also no legal requirement for a physician's prescription. This situation began to change early in the 1900s, when the federal government stepped in to protect consumers and to regulate the pharmaceutical industry. The states, too, established practice acts to regulate the dispensing and administration of drugs.

Federal Laws

Federal regulation of drugs was initially intended to protect consumers from harmful, impure, or unsafe drugs. Thus, when the Pure Food and Drug Act was passed in 1906, it set standards for quality and required the proper labeling of drugs. In 1938, the federal government began to address drug effectiveness. It passed the Food, Drug, and Cosmetic Act, which required animal testing of drugs. Thus, prior to selling a new drug, pharmaceutical companies had to apply for approval to market a drug, and that approval was contingent on proof that the drug was effective on animals. The Durham-Humphrey Amendments to the Food, Drug, and Cosmetic Act were passed in 1951. These amendments required a physician's order to dispense certain drugs, called **prescription drugs,** and established an over-the-counter **(OTC)** category of drugs that did not require a prescription. Then, in 1970, the Controlled Substance Act was passed. It designated certain drugs as **controlled substances.** See Table 3–1 for a summary of federal drug laws.

Table 3–1 Federal Drug Laws

Pure Food and Drug Act (1906)
- required all drugs marketed in the United States to meet minimal standards of uniform strength, purity, and quality
- required that preparations containing morphine be labeled
- established two references of officially approved drugs: the *United States Pharmacopoeia* (*USP*) and the *National Formulary* (*NF*)*

Federal Food, Drug, and Cosmetic Act (1938; Amended in 1951 and 1965)
- established the Food and Drug Administration (FDA)
- established specific regulations regarding warning labels on preparations, e.g., cautions about a drug's capacity to cause drowsiness or become habit-forming
- stated that both prescription and nonprescription drugs must be effective and safe
- stated that all labels must be accurate and include the generic name
- required FDA approval of all new drugs
- designated which drugs could be sold over-the-counter (OTC), i.e., without a prescription

Controlled Substances Act (1970)
- established the Drug Enforcement Agency (DEA)
- set tighter controls on drugs capable of being abused (controlled substances), e.g., depressants, stimulants, and narcotics
- required stricter security controls for anyone (physicians, pharmacists, hospitals) who dispenses, receives, sells, or destroys controlled substances
- set limits on the use of prescriptions: established guidelines for the number of times a drug can be prescribed in a period of time, and set rules on which preparations may be prescribed over the telephone to the pharmacy
- required that each prescriber register with the DEA, obtaining a DEA number to be used on prescriptions
- identified abusable and addicting drugs, classifying them into schedules according to the degree of danger

*These two publications have since been combined and are referred to as the *USP/NF*.

Table 3–2 Schedules of Controlled Substances

Schedule	Examples
C-I	Heroin, LSD, PCP, marijuana
C-II	Alfentanyl, opium, cocaine, codeine, morphine
C-III	Anabolic steroids, products with low amounts of codeine
C-IV	Diazepam, lorazepam, phenobarbital
C-V	Many antitussive and antidiarrheal agents

The Controlled Substances Act of 1970 established classifications, known as schedules, of drugs that had potential for abuse. Five schedules (Table 3–2) were determined, based on the level of abuse and dependence potential and on appropriate medical uses for the drug. Drugs such as LSD are listed on the C-I schedule; they have high abuse potential and no accepted medical use. Controlled substances from the C-II schedule have high abuse potential, but also have accepted medical uses. C-II controlled substances that are frequently used in surgery include alfentanyl, cocaine, and morphine. Drugs listed as C-III have moderate abuse potential, while drugs on schedules C-IV and C-V have low abuse potential.

The **Drug Enforcement Agency** (**DEA**) was established to enforce the Controlled Substances Act. It sets standards for handling controlled substances and has the legal authority to enforce those standards. Institutional policies and procedures for storing and handling controlled substances must comply with DEA standards, and documentation requirements must be strictly followed. When hospitals administer **narcotics,** for example, they must keep careful records of the amount of drug used as well as the date, the patient, the person administering the drug, and the person obtaining it.

State Practice Acts

State laws known as *practice acts* govern ordering, dispensing, and administration of medications. Such laws vary from state to state. For example, state laws regulate who—physicians, physician assistants, nurse practitioners—may prescribe drugs. They also regulate pharmacy practices, specifying how drugs are to be dispensed and by whom (usually a licensed pharmacist). Drug substitution laws, for example, specify if a pharmacist may automatically substitute a generic equivalent for a prescribed drug if not indicated otherwise.

Physicians can "lend" or delegate some of their functions to others. For example, the surgical technologist functions as a "physician extender"—an extra pair of hands, so to speak. As such, he or she performs drug-handling and administration duties under the delegatory power of the physician. Each state controls the limits of this delegatory power through the Medical Licensing Board.

☞ As a surgical technologist, you should be knowledgeable about the medication handling and administration laws in your own state. State practice acts are public information; this means you can read these acts yourself in order to be correctly informed. This is important because the delegatory power and its interpretations differ from state to state. For instance, many people believe that only nurses may administer medications to patients. However, in many states, credentialed allied health professionals such as perfusionists, respiratory therapists, and medical assistants routinely administer medications legally. The surgical technologists must have direct knowledge of, and function within, the legal standards of medication administration determined by the state in which they practice.

Local Policies

When state laws do not specifically address the practice of surgical technology, published institutional policies should be used to determine the scope of practice. The role of the surgical technologist in drug handling is usually specified in institutional policies, which have local authority. The surgical technologist must be thoroughly familiar with medication administration policies and closely adhere to their stated limits. If current policies are outdated, or do not reflect the scope of practice appropriate to the education and expertise of the surgical technologist, the institution should revise or update them as appropriate. The surgical technologist's job description may also contain relevant information regarding medication handling and administration.

☞ Under no circumstances should a surgical technologist exceed the limits of the facility's published job description. These job descriptions are subject to revision, as needed, to reflect current practice standards.

Drug Development

Prior to legal regulation, drugs could be manufactured, sold, and administered without scientific proof of safety, quality, or effectiveness. Today, all drugs must undergo stringent testing and provide proof of safety and effectiveness before release. The federal **Food and Drug Administration** (**FDA**) regulates the pharmaceutical industry, ensuring that basic standards are followed. To do this, the FDA inspects the facilities where drugs are made, reviews new drug applications, investigates and removes unsafe drugs from the market, and requires proper labeling of drugs.

Phases of Drug Testing

Pharmaceutical companies are continually developing new drugs, and each new drug must undergo required testing prior to FDA approval. This testing is an extensive process. All new drugs are first tested on animals to determine if the drug is safe to administer to humans. At least two species of mammals, of both genders, must be used for this initial stage of drug testing. During this process, researchers look for toxic effects and determine safe dosage levels. Once the drug has proven safe in animals, the drug company applies to the FDA for permission to begin human testing. There are four phases of human testing, as summarized in Table 3–3.

Phase I: Clinical Pharmacology   In the clinical pharmacology phase, the new drug is given to healthy volunteers, usually males between the ages of 18 and 45. This phase is used to determine the dose level for symptoms of drug toxicity in humans.

Phase II: Clinical Investigation   In the clinical investigation phase, the drug is given to limited numbers of patients presenting with the disease or condition the drug was developed to treat. The clinical investigation phase is used to establish drug effectiveness and to determine optimum dosage and dose range.

Phase III: Clinical Trials   In the clinical trial phase researchers continue to note drug effectiveness, safety, and side effects in large studies. In this phase, which begins only if no serious side effects occur in Phase II, the new drug is given to hundreds or thousands of patients, usually in large medical research facilities. The drug's effectiveness is verified and its actions are characterized by various types of scientific studies. Several kinds of studies may be conducted. For instance, in *double-blind studies,* half of the testing group receives the drug and the other half receives an inactive substance called a placebo. Neither the subject patients nor the prescribing physicians

Table 3–3   Phases of Human Drug Testing

Phase	Purpose
Phase I: Clinical Pharmacology	Determine toxicity levels
Phase II: Clinical Investigation	Establish effectiveness; determine optimum dosage and dose range
Phase III: Clinical Trials	Assess drug effectiveness
Phase IV: Post-marketing Study	Continue study and documentation

know which group received the placebo until the study has been completed. The results of these and other studies must be thoroughly documented.

Phase IV: Post-marketing Study   The post-marketing study phase occurs after the drug is released for use in treatment of the specified condition. In this phase the drug company continues to monitor the drug, gathering results from prescribing physicians. This continuing evaluation of the drug includes results from those patients excluded from the previous phases, such as pregnant patients and the elderly. These data must be gathered, analyzed, and reported to the FDA in order to document the drug's safety and effectiveness comprehensively.

Marketing

During development, the drug company assigns a generic name to the new drug. Later, it selects a company trade name, which it uses for marketing purposes once the drug gains FDA approval. The ***United States Pharmacopoeia and National Formulary (USP/NF)*** assigns an official name to the new drug; this is usually the generic name. Once a drug has been approved for release, the pharmaceutical company responsible for the drug's development has exclusive rights to market that drug under its trade name for seventeen years. This process allows the drug company to recover development costs. After these exclusive rights have expired, other companies may begin to market a generic equivalent with a different trade name.

Drug References

When a drug has been approved for use, the pharmaceutical company must publish comprehensive information regarding the drug. This information must appear in package inserts and in compiled reference works. In addition, many drug information resources are available to medical, nursing, and allied health professionals. There are dozens of textbooks on pharmacology and various specialty areas within that science. Moreover, several pharmacology resources are expressly designed for use in clinical practice. Each surgery department should have such references readily available to the staff.

Physician's Desk Reference

One of the most frequently used pharmacology resources is the *Physician's Desk Reference,* or ***PDR.*** It provides easy access to information about drugs used in medical and surgical practice. The *PDR* is divided into six color-coded sections:

1. A list of drug manufacturers
2. An index of brand and generic drug names
3. A list of drugs by prescribing category
4. A photographic identification section
5. A product information section
6. A section on diagnostic agents.

The product information section, which is the largest part of the book, contains manufacturer's information on approximately 3,000 drugs. Drugs are listed alphabetically by manufacturer. Each entry includes data on **indications,** effects, dosage, administration routes, methods, and frequency. It also includes warnings regarding side effects and **contraindications.** The *PDR* is revised annually.

☞ The information presented in the *PDR* is the same as that found in the manufacturer's package insert. Students may easily obtain package inserts for drugs used in surgery. You can get them as medications are opened or from the pharmacy at your clinical site.

United States Pharmacopoeia and National Formulary

The *USP/NF* is the official drug list recognized by the United States government. It is actually two publications—the Pharmacopoeia and the Formulary—combined into one volume. The *USP/NF* lists standards for drug quality, safety, and effectiveness; it also contains information on the physical and chemical characteristics of listed drugs. Used primarily by drug companies and pharmacists, the *USP/NF* is revised every five years. It is prepared under the supervision of a national committee of pharmacists, pharmacologists, physicians, chemists, biologists, and other scientific professionals. The *United States Pharmacopoeia Dispensing Information (USPDI)* is a related clinical reference divided into two volumes—one for health care providers and one for patients.

Hospital Pharmacist

Another valuable source of information on drugs is the clinical pharmacist. Consulting and educating has become an important part of pharmacy practice. The pharmacist is consulted when any question arises regarding medications, especially newly released drugs.

Data Bases

A vast amount of information regarding medications, their proper use, possible drug side effects and interactions, and other important clinical considerations is available via computer. Data bases, such as *Micromedex,* are helpful tools that medical professionals use to access current pharmacologic information. The Internet also allows you to access drug information. Helpful Internet addresses include:

The National Institute of Health (NIH) at http://www.nih.gov/
The National Library of Medicine at http://www.nlm.nih.gov/
The Pharmaceutical Information Network at http://pharminfo.com/

Other drug resource material is easily accessible by computer, including the *USPDI, PDR,* current journal articles, and manufacturer's bulletins.

Summary

Prior to federal regulation in the United States, drugs could be manufactured and sold without proof of safety or effectiveness. In the twentieth century the federal government enacted several laws to ensure consumer safety and regulate the pharmaceutical industry. The FDA is the federal agency responsible for monitoring drug development, manufacturing, and marketing. New drugs must be thoroughly tested prior to approval for release by the FDA. When a new drug is released for use, the manufacturer provides comprehensive information about the drug. Many drug information resources are available. Surgical technologists should become familiar with pharmacology reference materials available in their own clinical facilities. It is also important to use drug information resources to stay up-to-date on new drugs.

REVIEW

1. How does the federal government regulate drugs?

2. How is medication administration regulated in your state?

3. How is medication handling and administration specified in one of your school's clinical affiliates?

4. What is the role of the FDA in drug regulation? How does the DEA affect clinical practice?

5. What is the purpose of each phase of drug testing?

6. Use at least two different clinical drug references to look up indications for and side effects of the following drugs: (**a**) epinephrine; (**b**) lidocaine; (**c**) mannitol; (**d**) ranitidine.

CHAPTER 4

Drug Administration

OBJECTIVES

Upon completion of this chapter you should be able to:

1 Describe the role of the surgical technologist in medication administration.
2 Explain the five "rights" of medication administration.
3 Describe the steps of medication identification.
4 Discuss aseptic techniques for delivery of medications to the sterile field.
5 List methods for labeling drugs on the sterile back table.
6 Identify supplies used in medication administration in surgery.

KEY TERMS

Contamination Transmission of microorganisms to a sterile field or items.

Negligence Failure to do something an ordinarily prudent person would do in a certain situation; doing something that an ordinarily prudent person would not do.

The role of the surgical technologist in medication administration varies from state to state and differs from facility to facility. As a surgical technologist, you should have first-hand knowledge of drug administration legislation in your state. Institutional policies and procedures regarding medication handling and administration should be clearly understood as well. All staff members have a duty to be familiar with and adhere to established medication policies and procedures. Handling medications is a critical function in the surgical technologist's job description. Several different types of drugs are obtained and passed to the surgeon routinely during a procedure, and the surgical technologist must be knowledgeable regarding such drugs.

☞ The limits of legal authority for the surgical technologist to perform the indicated roles described in this text are controlled by each state through its statutes, case law, regulatory law, attorney general opinions, and medical licensing boards. Discussion of these sources of law is beyond the scope of this text. Except as otherwise noted, this book describes the general practice of surgical technology in the United States, not the legal authority for such practice. It is the surgical technologist's responsibility to consult the limitations in his/her area on acts described in this book.

Surgical Technologist's Role in Drug Administration

Administration of drugs from the sterile field is a team effort. Routinely, medications used in surgery will be obtained by the *circulator,* passed to the *scrub,* and then to the surgeon for administration. Each team member is responsible for accurate identification of drugs used during a surgical procedure.

Circulating Role

The surgical technologist in the circulating role obtains medications as specified on the surgeon's preference card, then delivers those medications to the sterile field as needed. The circulator must maintain strict asepsis when transferring medications to the scrub person. All medications must be properly identified, both by the scrub and by the circulator. The circulator is responsible for documenting all medications used from the sterile field according to institutional policy.

Scrub Role

The surgical technologist in the scrub role accepts medications from the circulator, properly labels (Fig. 4–1) those medications, then passes them to the surgeon as requested. Accurate identification and labeling of drugs accepted into the sterile field is crucial. If medications are not clearly identified, they should be discarded and a new dose should be obtained. This is essential to avoid possible drug administration error.

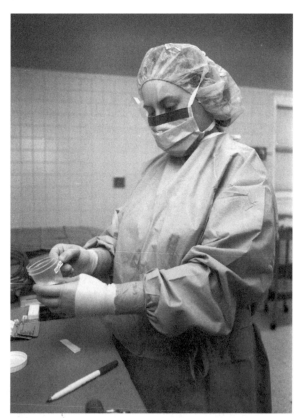

Figure 4–1 The scrubbed surgical technologist labels medications immediately.

The "Five Rights" of Medication Administration

To help prevent medication errors, the "Five Rights" of medication administration have been established (Table 4–1). Team members must work together to ensure that the right drug is given in the right dose, by the right route, to the right patient, at the right time.

Right Drug

Drugs that are routinely needed on the sterile field during a procedure should be clearly specified on the surgeon's preference card by the surgery staff (surgical technologists; registered nurses). The information stated on the preference card must be accurate, including correct spelling and strength. Handwritten preference cards (Fig. 4–2), must be written legibly to avoid confusion. Preference cards should be updated as needed to reflect any changes in routine medications. Additional drugs are obtained in response to verbal orders by the surgeon during the procedure.

When any drug is delivered to the sterile back table, it must be carefully identified, then labeled accurately. The scrub person always states the name and strength of the drug aloud as he or she hands it to the surgeon; this practice serves as confirmation that the medication is correct. All empty medication vials and bottles should be kept in the room during the procedure as evidence that the proper medication has been delivered to the field.

Right Dose

The dose of a drug includes both its amount (volume) and its strength (concentration). You might see, for instance, an order for 30 mL (amount) of 0.5% (strength) lidocaine with epinephrine on a physician's preference card. This information must be clearly specified and clearly understood. It's especially important when the drug must be mixed or diluted on the sterile back table. Suppose, for example, a surgeon requests $\frac{1}{2}$ cc of 1% phenylephrine (Neosynephrine)

Table 4–1 **Five Rights of Medication Administration**

- Right Drug—**What** drug is required?
- Right Dose—**How much** of the drug is required in **what concentration?**
- Right Route—**How** will the drug be administered?
- Right Patient—**Who** will receive the drug?
- Right Time—**When** will the drug be administered?

Surgeon: Dr. Ferguson	Procedure: Excision skin lesions (local)
Glove size: 7 1/2 Skin prep: Betadine	Position of patient: According to lesions Drapes: towels—drape sheets If face, split sheet and turban drape
SUTURES AND NEEDLES	INSTRUMENTS AND EQUIPMENT
Ties: Peritoneum: Fascia: Sub-cu: Skin: 5-0 Dermalon > have in room 6-0 mild chromic > do not open Retention: Other:	Basic: Small dissecting set Special: 4x8 (RP's) sponges cautery pencil c̄ needle tip #11 knife blade CD player
Dressings: steri-strips	Local anesthetic: 1% lidocaine c̄ epinephrine 5cc syringe #18 g. and #25 g. needles

Figure 4–2 Handwritten surgeon's preference card showing medication needed for procedure.

diluted in 20 cc of saline. Further suppose that phenylephrine is available in 1-cc vials. If the entire 1-cc vial is mixed with the correct amount (20 cc) of saline and dispensed to the sterile field, the dosage of phenylephrine administered will be *twice* the desired dose.

Written protocols may be instituted and posted to eliminate common confusions about some medications. Take heparin, for instance. During insertion of a venous access port, different strengths of heparin (an anticoagulant) may be needed: 100 units per milliliter and 10 units per milliliter may be used, each concentration with a specific purpose. In this case, a department routine or protocol for heparin dosages in venous access procedures may be established to minimize the potential for error.

Right Route

Most drugs administered in surgery are given intravenously, usually by the anesthesia provider. Drugs may also be injected or applied topically by the surgeon. Different routes require different preparations and concentrations. The preference card should state administration route clearly, so that the proper form of the drug for a particular route may be obtained.

Right Patient

Although the possibility of administering a drug to the wrong patient in surgery is remote, it is not unknown. Thus caution must be exercised to avoid errors. All surgical patients must be accurately identified prior to transport into the operating room. This identification should also include important information about the patient. For example, any history of drug allergies should be noted. In addition, the surgical procedure and operating surgeon should be verified, and the preference card containing medication orders for that specific procedure should be kept available in the operating room.

Right Time

Intraoperatively, drugs are usually ordered for one-time administration only. The purpose of the drug often indicates the timing of administration. If, for example, 1% lidocaine with epinephrine is listed on the preference card for a local anesthetic, it will be administered prior to incision. Some routine medications (e.g., contrast media for cholangiography, antibiotics for irrigation, or anesthetic agents for postoperative pain block) are obtained and labeled during case setup, then passed at the appropriate time. Other medications may be obtained and passed from the sterile back table as soon as requested by the surgeon.

Medication Identification

Both the scrub and circulator are responsible for correctly identifying medications delivered to and used from the sterile field. This dual responsibility minimizes the potential for errors in medication administration, as does the use of a logical series of steps to properly identify drugs. The first step in medication identification is to read the label on the medicine container (Fig. 4–3). The team member obtaining the drug reads the label initially, then checks the container for cracks or discolored contents. If there is any doubt as to the integrity of the container, the medication should not be used. Rather, it should be returned to the pharmacy with a note indicating the specific concern. The medication label contains important information about the drug, as Table 4–2 shows. The most crucial information is the drug name—both generic and trade—the strength, the amount, and the expiration date. The circulator reads this label information aloud just prior to delivery to the sterile field, then shows the label to the scrub person (Fig. 4–4). Finally, the scrub repeats the label information aloud to confirm

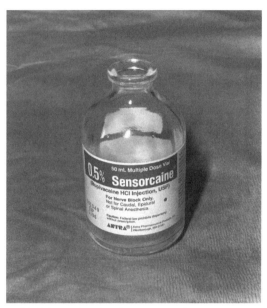

Figure 4–3 Medication label. (Reproduced with permission of Astra USA, Inc., 50 Otis Street, Westborough, MA 01581-4500.)

the correct drug. The drug should be delivered to the sterile field only after the steps described have been completed.

Delivery to the Sterile Field

Principles of asepsis must be followed when delivering and receiving medications into the sterile field. Medications frequently used from the sterile back

Table 4–2   A Sample Medication Label

Type of Information	Example
Name (brand and generic)	Sensorcaine (bupivicaine HCl)
Strength	0.5%
Amount	50 mL
Expiration date	01/99
Administration route	Injection
Manufacturer	Astra
Storage directions	Store at room temperature
Warnings or precautions	Federal law prohibits dispensing without prescription
Lot number	1234567
Schedule (C-I to C-V)*	

* Only if drug is a controlled substance.

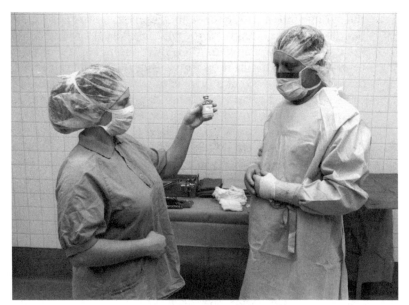

Figure 4–4 The circulator shows a drug label to the scrub.

table are packaged in different types of containers (Fig. 4–5). One of the most common containers is a glass or plastic vial with a rubber stopper encased in a metal cap. The metal cap is peeled away so that the circulator can draw up the drug (if in liquid form) with a syringe and needle and then empty the contents of

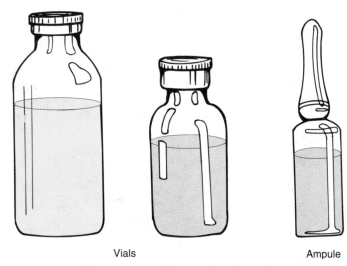

Vials   Ampule

Figure 4–5 Medication vials and ampule.

the syringe into a sterile medicine cup held by the scrub. The circulator should handle only the outside of the vial and should not touch the rubber stopper unless it is being removed. Alternatively, the circulator may hold the vial in an inverted position while the scrub withdraws the drug from the vial with a syringe and needle (Fig. 4–6). If a drug is in powder form in a vial, the circulator must reconstitute it with an appropriate liquid, such as saline (NaCl) solution, withdraw the resulting liquid, and deliver it to the sterile field as described above. If a syringe is used to draw up and inject the reconstituting agent and to withdraw the mixture, care must be taken not to touch the sides of the plunger (Fig. 4–7). If the plunger is touched by unsterile hands, it contaminates the inside of the barrel as it moves down the barrel when injecting. If the drug mixture is then drawn into the syringe barrel, it becomes contaminated as well.

In some cases, the rubber top of a vial may be removed aseptically and the solution poured directly into a medicine cup (Fig. 4–8). If the stopper is removed for pouring, care must be taken to avoid contact with the lip of the vial, which must remain sterile. Sterile disposable spouts are commercially available to facilitate sterile delivery of medications contained in vials and in bags of intravenous solution. Medications may be added to a bag of intravenous solution, such as a gram of an antibiotic into 1000 cc of normal saline, and disposable spouts may be used to deliver the solution to the sterile field aseptically.

Some medications are available in an ampule, a sealed glass container with a narrowed neck. The top of an ampule is broken off at the neck and a sterile needle is inserted to withdraw the medication. Special care should be used when breaking the glass ampule, as glass may cut unprotected hands (Fig. 4–9). Some glass ampules also come packaged sterile for use on the back table, such as the liquid

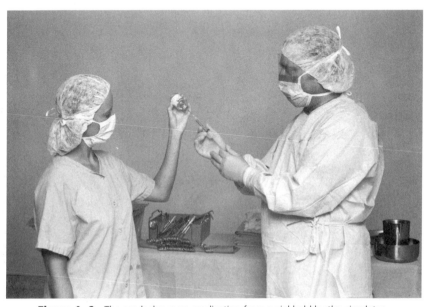

Figure 4–6 The scrub draws up medication from a vial held by the circulator.

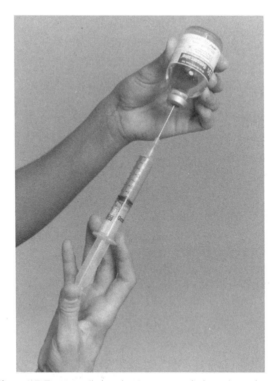

Figure 4–7 Unsterile hands must not touch the syringe plunger.

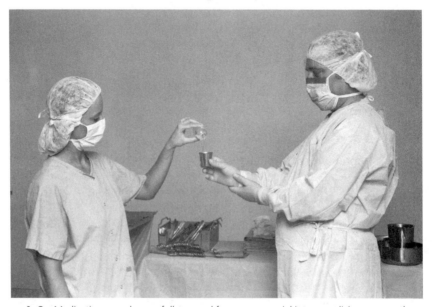

Figure 4–8 Medications may be carefully poured from an open vial into a medicine cup or other container.

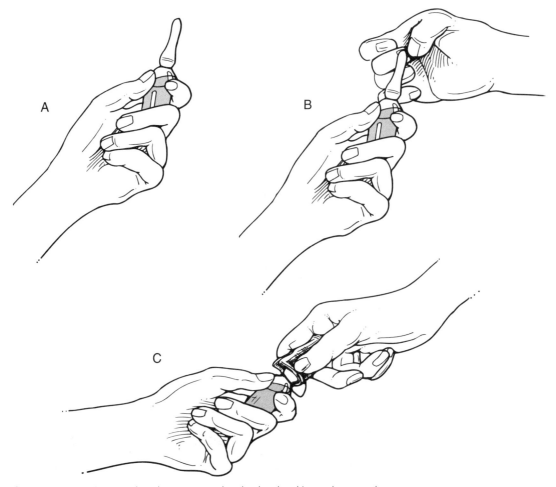

Figure 4–9   Caution must be taken to protect hands when breaking a glass ampule.

component used to make methyl methacrylate (bone cement). Once again, care must be taken to protect the gloved hands. After the ampule is broken, the sponge or wrapper used to protect the hands should be discarded from the sterile field to avoid accidental transfer of glass particles into the surgical wound.

If medication is contained in a pour bottle (as seen in antibiotic irrigation prepared in the pharmacy), the cap should be lifted straight up and off, and the entire contents poured immediately. Unused portions should not be saved for later use, as sterility cannot be assured. If the bottle is recapped, its contents are considered unsterile due to potential contamination of the bottle lip during replacement of the cap.

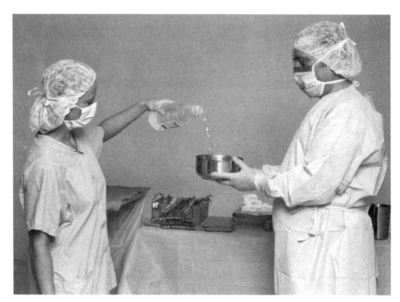

Figure 4–10 The circulator must not lean over the sterile field when delivering medications or solutions.

The circulator must take care not to lean over the sterile field (Fig. 4–10) when delivering medications or solutions to avoid potential **contamination.** The scrub should hold containers away from the sterile table or place containers at the table edge. Several different types of containers are available to store medications and solutions on the sterile back table (Fig. 4–11). Medicine cups, pitchers, basins, or syringes may be used, depending on the volume of medication needed.

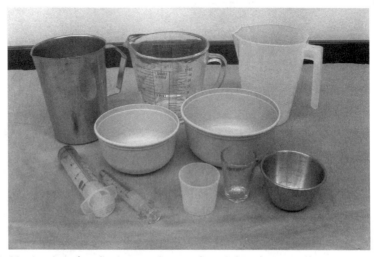

Figure 4–11 A variety of medication containers, such as pitchers, basins, medicine cups, or syringes may be used on the sterile back table.

Medication Labeling

Once a medication has been delivered to the sterile back table, it must be labeled immediately. Most drugs used from the sterile field are clear in color; thus, they are easily confused if not clearly marked. There are many different methods of labeling medications on the sterile back table, only a few of which are described as examples (Fig. 4–12). Sterile solution markers may be placed inside pitchers or basins. A skin marking pen may be used to indicate the drug name on a sterile label, which is then placed on a syringe or other container. If sterile labels are not available, Steri-strip bandages may be used. Preprinted drug labels are also available in some locations.

In some instances, other items already opened on the table may be used to label drugs creatively. For example, during a cholangiogram, you need two syringes—a syringe containing saline and a syringe containing contrast medium. You might place a silk tie (ligature) around the syringe containing contrast medium to differentiate it from saline. Regardless of the labeling method employed, proper identification of all medications on the sterile field will help prevent administration errors.

Occasionally, the scrub person may be replaced during a procedure (e.g., shift change or lunch relief). All medications must be plainly labeled and reported to the new scrub person. If there is any doubt as to the identity of a solution, it must be discarded and new medication must be obtained.

Improper or inadequate labeling of drugs may be considered negligent. **Negligence** is defined in the Miller–Keane *Encyclopedia and Dictionary of Medicine,*

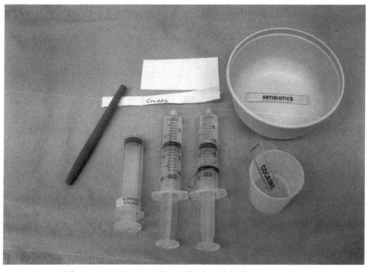

Figure 4–12   Sample sterile drug labeling methods.

Nursing and Allied Health as "failure to do something that a reasonable person of ordinary prudence would do in a situation or the doing of something that such a person would not do." By this definition, it is "reasonable" to expect that the correct drug will be obtained, identified, and passed to the surgeon . . . and that a "prudent" person will perform these duties. This means that reason and prudence are everyone's responsibility, whatever the situation. This isn't always easy. The rapid pace of events in surgery often pressures team members to accomplish difficult tasks in a hurry. However, the process of medication identification should never be compromised; nor should staff become complacent about routine medications. If a question or doubt arises regarding a medication, it must be clarified and resolved. If the medication seems wrong, or the dose appears to be incorrect, verify it with the physician before using it. It is better to be certain about the drug—even if it means provoking the surgeon—than to make an error and thus cause harm to the patient.

☞ Do not be embarrassed to admit ignorance or confusion. And always admit an outright error. Honesty and integrity are vital characteristics in health care professionals. If you make a medication error, acknowledge it at once, so that corrective measures may be taken. Notify the surgeon immediately. Then follow institutional policy. Usually, when a medication error occurs, the unit supervisor is notified and an incident or occurrence report is completed. Above all, immediate action is taken to correct the error, thus ensuring patient safety.

Special caution is required when handling controlled substances in surgery. Local policies regarding handling of controlled substances must be in compliance with federal law (see Chapter 3); thus, they must be understood and followed by all staff members. For example, cocaine is a schedule C-II drug frequently used for topical anesthesia in surgery. If needed for a particular procedure, cocaine will be obtained immediately prior to use, and never left unattended. Any cocaine remaining at the end of the procedure must be rendered useless—usually by dilution with large amounts of water—then discarded. The dilution and disposal of any controlled substance should be witnessed by at least two team members.

Supplies

Syringes and needles are frequently used to administer medications. Various types and sizes of syringes are used to draw up and inject drugs (Fig. 4–13). Syringes are usually made of plastic, but glass syringes may be used occasionally. The most common type of syringe used in surgery is the Luer-loc tip, which has a screw-type locking mechanism used to securely attach a needle. Plain-tip

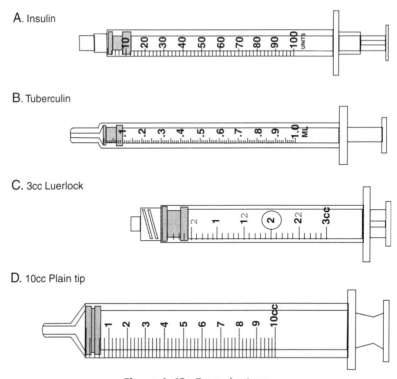

Figure 4–13 Types of syringes.

or slip-tip syringes are also available, but these are used for specific purposes. For example, a plain-tip syringe may be attached to a spinal needle for subclavian venipuncture during a venous access procedure. Some syringes have a finger-control attachment to provide ease of motion when injecting. Syringes also come in various sizes. Sizes of syringes routinely used in surgery range from 1 cc to 60 cc. The barrel of the syringe is marked to indicate the amount of medication contained in the syringe.

Special syringes are available for particular purposes. For example, a tubex syringe has a metal or plastic device used to accommodate a carpule of medication for injection (such as lidocaine or heparin). The glass medication carpule has a rubber cap that is penetrated by a special needle attached to the tubex syringe (Fig. 4–14).

Many types of needles are used in surgery to draw up and administer drugs. Needles vary in diameter (gauge) and length (measured in inches). The larger the gauge of needle, the smaller the diameter of the lumen (inside channel). Most needles used in surgery are disposable and are color-coded by size at the plastic hub (Fig. 4–15) for ease in identification. Reusable, all-metal, needles are available with the gauge engraved on the hub. Sizes of needles routinely used in surgery range from tiny 30-gauge needles (used in ophthalmology) to larger 18-

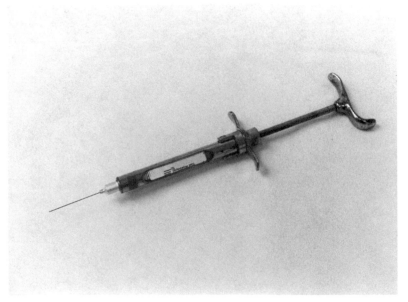

Figure 4–14 A tubex syringe, glass carpule, and needle.

gauge needles (used to draw up drugs). The most common needle length used is $1\frac{1}{2}$ inches. Longer needles, called spinal needles, may be used for specific purposes, such as aspiration of cysts.

☞ Universal Precautions state that used needles must never be recapped, as most needle puncture injuries are the result of attempting to recap a used needle. However, if a needle must be recapped, you should use a one-handed technique (Fig. 4–16) or a recapping device intended for that purpose.

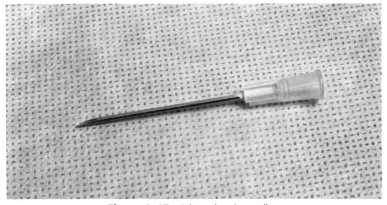

Figure 4–15 A hypodermic needle.

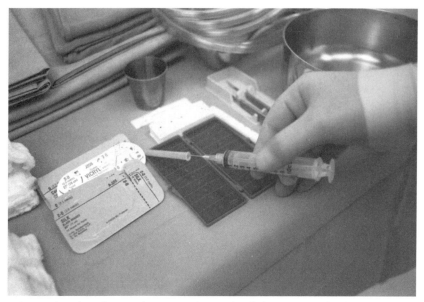

Figure 4–16 If used needles must be recapped, a one-handed recapping technique may be used.

Summary

The role of the surgical technologist in medication administration tends to vary from institution to institution. Each facility's established policies and procedures should always be understood and scrupulously followed. In addition, the surgical technologist must be aware of state regulations regarding specific practices.

Application of the five "rights" of medication administration will reduce the potential for drug errors. The surgical technologist in the scrub role must never accept a medication without properly identifying it. Aseptic technique must be used when delivering or accepting drugs into the sterile field. Accurate and immediate labeling of drugs on the sterile back table is required to minimize potential for errors.

REVIEW

1. How is drug administration handled in surgery at your clinical facility?

2. Give examples of applications of the five "rights" of medication administration in surgery.

3. List the logical steps necessary to accurately identify drugs in surgery.

4. Describe proper aseptic technique when delivering drugs to the sterile field.

5. What methods are used to label drugs on the sterile field at your clinical facility?

UNIT **TWO**

Applied Surgical Pharmacology

Many medications are used in surgery each day. This unit provides an introduction to the medications you'll frequently encounter as a surgical technologist. We'll look at antibiotics, diagnostic agents, diuretics, gastric drugs, and hormones. We'll also examine drugs that affect blood coagulation and drugs used as ophthalmic agents. To understand these drugs, you'll need to be familiar with some basic anatomy and physiology, so we'll review some of those principles, as well. Thus, once you know the generic and brand names of common surgical drugs and their categories, you'll recognize their purposes, action, administration, routes, and proper handling in order to provide safe patient care.

CHAPTER **5**

Antibiotics

OBJECTIVES

Upon completion of this chapter you should be able to:

1 Define terminology related to antimicrobial therapy.
2 Discuss the purpose of antibiotic therapy in surgery.
3 Describe various ways in which antimicrobials work.
4 Discuss antibiotic resistance.
5 List categories of antibiotics used in surgery and give examples of each.
6 Use drug resources to gather pertinent information on antibiotics.

KEY TERMS

Aerobic Ability to grow in the presence of oxygen.

Anaerobic Ability to grow in the absence of oxygen.

Bactericidal Bacteria-killing; destructive to bacteria.

Bacteriostatic Bacteria-stopping; inhibiting the growth of bacteria.

Culture and sensitivity (C&S) Series of tests used to identify pathogenic microorganisms and determine their susceptibility to various antibiotics.

Gram-positive Type of bacteria whose cell walls retain the primary purple dye used in gram staining.

Gram-negative Type of bacteria whose cell walls take on the secondary red counterstain used in gram staining.

MRSA Methicillin-resistant *Staphylococcus aureus;* a strain of staph bacteria that is unresponsive to the antibiotic methicillin.

Prophylaxis Prevention; preventive treatment.

TB Tubercle bacillus, or tuberculosis.

VRE Vancomycin-resistant enterococci; strains of the Streptococcus family of bacteria (normally found in the digestive tract) that are unresponsive to the antibiotic vancomycin.

Before the discovery of antimicrobial agents, surgical patients often died from infections of various kinds. Surgical procedures, such as amputations, were quite dangerous in themselves. However the most common danger was postoperative wound infections. Even if patients survived surgery, the resulting wound infection was often fatal. Today, however, many antimicrobial agents are available. They are used (1) to prevent and (2) to treat infections caused by pathogenic (disease-causing) microorganisms. The term *antimicrobial* applies to several categories of agents: These include antivirals, antibacterials, antiprotozoals, antifungals, and antiparasitics. In surgery, however, the only antimicrobial agents routinely used are antibacterials, commonly referred to as *antibiotics.*

Antibiotics are natural chemicals (or *metabolites*) produced by microorganisms, these natural chemicals may be altered in the chemical laboratory to produce semisynthetic antibiotics. Approximately 85% of the antibiotics currently available are produced by actinomycetes—bacteria that resemble fungi because of their filamentous projections. Other antibiotics, such as the penicillins, are derived from fungi.

Antibiotics are given both preoperatively and intraoperatively for **prophylaxis**—i.e., prevention—of postoperative wound infections. They may also be prescribed postoperatively. Postoperative wound infections are potential complications of every surgical intervention because any such procedure penetrates the body's first line of defense, the skin. Postoperative wound infections may range from minor to serious; they may even be deadly, depending on several factors. Antibiotics do not take the place of aseptic technique. Rather, antibiotics are adjuncts that assist the patient's own defenses to prevent—or diminish the severity of—postoperative wound infections.

Microbiology Review

Postoperative wound infections are caused by the introduction of pathogenic microorganisms into a susceptible host. Pathogenic microorganisms may be exogenous or endogenous. That is, they may come from outside the patient (exogenous) or they may come from the patient's own bacteria (endogenous). For example, among the most common causative agents of postoperative wound infections are bacteria known as *Staphylococcus aureus,* which are normally resident on human skin. Other bacteria, such as the mycobacteria that cause tuberculosis, are not usually resident in the human body. Many factors influence host susceptibility to an infection, including general health, nutritional status, operative site, and length of surgical procedure.

If a postoperative wound infection occurs, treatment requires identification of the causative microorganism and selection of an appropriate antimicrobial agent. Pathogenic microorganisms causing postoperative wound infections are identified by several methods. Common methods used to identify pathogens include **culture and sensitivity (C&S)** and gram staining. Acid-fast stains can be used to identify such particular organisms as the **tubercle bacillus (TB).** To perform culture and sensitivity, a fluid or tissue specimen is obtained with a swab from the infection site, then placed in one or more culture tubes for transport to the microbiology laboratory. [Separate culture tubes are available for **aerobic** (in oxygen) and **anaerobic** (lacking oxygen) testing.] In the laboratory, the culture swab is used to spread the fluid sample onto nutrient agar and differential (distinguishing) media in petri dishes called *plates.* This process is called *inoculation.* The inoculated plates are incubated for 24–48 hours, after which they can be examined for microbial growth.

Once the microbe has been isolated, it is cultured again so it can be exposed to different antibiotics. This process of successive exposure to antibiotics to determine which agent is most effective against it is called *sensitivity testing.*

☞ Computers and miniaturized reaction containers allow lab personnel to identify causative microbes more easily. Computers and miniaturization have also been used to provide rapid sensitivity testing.

When the causative microorganism is identified and tested for antibiotic sensitivity, the appropriate therapy can be initiated. Often, however, a broad-spectrum antibiotic is prescribed to begin treatment while awaiting the results of C&S testing. Occasionally, during a surgical procedure such as an incision and

INSIGHT 5-1 | GRAM STAINING

Gram staining is a differential staining procedure, which means it's used to distinguish between two types of bacteria. The gram stain procedure was developed in 1884 and is still widely used today. A specimen containing the pathogenic microorganism to be identified is swabbed onto a slide and fixed. Crystal violet is applied first, staining all cells a bluish-purple. Gram's iodine is then applied to the slide as a mordant—an agent that increases the cell's affinity for the primary stain. The slide is then rinsed with acetone or alcohol, decolorizing the cells. Next, safranin—a red counterstain—is applied. Only cells that were decolorized pick up the red counterstain. The cell walls of gram-positive bacteria do not decolorize, remaining purple. Gram-negative bacteria lose the purple stain during decolorization, so they appear red or reddish-pink after application of safranin.

drainage (I&D), a sample of abscess fluid may be subjected to an immediate gram stain (see Insight 5–1).

This immediate test assists the physician in prescribing an initial course of antibiotic therapy. Gram staining is a way of distinguishing types of bacteria. In combination with morphology (the study of shapes), it can be used to identify many common bacteria. Table 5–1 lists microorganisms classified by gram stain and morphology.

To be effective, antimicrobial agents must act against pathogenic microorganisms without harming host cells. That is, they must target structures and functions in pathogenic microorganisms that differ from those of host cells. In

Table 5–1 Pathogenic Microorganisms by Gram Staining and Morphology

Gram-Positive	Gram-Negative
Cocci	
Staphylococcus aureus	*Neisseria meningitidis*
Streptococcus species	
Enterococci	
Rods (bacilli)	
Mycobacterium tuberculosis	*Klebsiella pneumoniae*
	Enterobacter
	Escherichia coli
	Pseudomonas aeruginosa
	Proteus
	Serratia
	Haemophilus influenzae

order to understand how antimicrobials work, then, we need to know what differences exist between pathogen and host cell structure.

Bacteria are one-celled organisms that don't have a fully developed nucleus. This means they are classified as *prokaryotes*. (A "karyote" is a nucleus. A *prokaryote* is an early, or "pre" nucleus.) Multicellular organisms, including fungi, plants, and animals, are classified as eukaryotes ("true" karyotes). Both prokaryotic and eukaryotic cells have a plasma membrane that encloses the cell and preserves its integrity. Thus it both protects the cell and regulates the movement of materials in and out of the cell. Prokaryotes differ from eukaryotes because they have a cell wall in addition to the plasma membrane. This cell wall provides a potential location for antibiotic therapy. (See Fig. 5–1.)

Prokaryotic cells also differ from eukaryotic cells in the structures responsible for protein synthesis—the *ribosomes*. These tiny structures assemble or synthesize proteins from amino acids. Both prokaryotes and eukaryotes have ribosomes, but prokaryotic ribosomes are smaller than eukaryotic ribosomes (Fig. 5–2). This size difference offers another avenue of action for antibiotics. That is, antibiotics that bind to the smaller bacterial ribosomes do not bind to the larger ribosomes of the eukaryotic host cells.

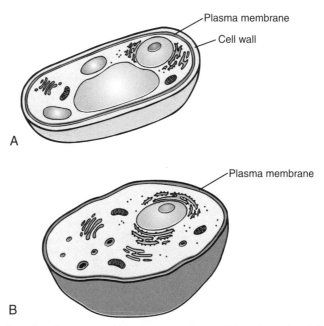

Figure 5–1 Eukaryotic cells are encased in a plasma membrane while prokaryotic cells have a cell wall in addition to a plasma membrane: (**A**) Prokaryotic cell; (**B**) eukaryotic cell.

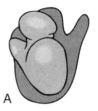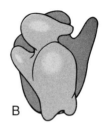

Figure 5–2 Prokaryotic (**A**) and eukaryotic (**B**) ribosomes differ in size.

A   B

Antimicrobial Action

Mechanisms and Types

Antimicrobial agents may work against pathogenic microorganisms by five different mechanisms, as summarized by Table 5–2. Some agents, such as cephalosporins, penicillins, vancomycin, and bacitracin, keep bacteria from synthesizing adequate cell walls. They can stop cell walls from forming or inhibit the synthesis process so the walls are too weak to maintain vital functions. Antibiotics such as aminoglycosides, erythromycins, and tetracyclines interfere with protein synthesis. This means they bind to prokaryotic ribosomes, thus preventing the assembly of critical proteins. Polymixins and some antifungal agents work by disrupting the bacterial cell wall membrane, causing leakage of materials necessary for cell function. A few agents, like quinolones and some antivirals, inhibit production of the nucleic acids (RNA or DNA) that are necessary for bacterial replication. Still other agents interfere with bacterial cell metabolism. Sulfonamides, for example, take the place of a vital substance needed to produce folic acid.

We classify antimicrobial agents as bactericidal or bacteriostatic. **Bactericidal** agents kill bacteria. These include agents such as the aminoglycosides, cephalosporins, and penicillins. **Bacteriostatic** agents inhibit bacterial growth, relying on the host's own immune system to take over once the pathogenic microorganism is suppressed. These include the erythromycins and tetracyclines. Antimicrobial agents are also classified by their *spectrum* of activity. A *broad-spectrum* antibiotic has a wide range of activity—usually against both gram-negative and gram-positive bacteria. *Narrow-spectrum* antibiotics have a smaller range of activity—often against only one category of microorganisms,

Table 5–2 **Methods of Antimicrobial Action**

Inhibit cell-wall synthesis
Interfere with protein synthesis
Alter cell wall membrane function
Inhibit production of nucleic acids (RNA or DNA)
Interfere with cell metabolism

gram-negative or gram-positive. *Limited-spectrum* antibiotics are effective against just one species of microorganism.

Antibiotic Resistance

Certain pathogenic microorganisms have developed an alarming capacity to resist antibiotics (see Insight 5–2). Known as *antibiotic resistance,* this capacity falls into three major categories:

- the microorganism may manufacture microbial enzymes that inactivate the antibiotic
- the agent may be prevented from reaching the target area
- the target area may be altered so that the agent is no longer effective.

INSIGHT 5–2 | **DEVELOPING AND SHARING ANTIBIOTIC RESISTANCE**

Microorganisms grow and divide rapidly so genetic material (DNA) is constantly replicated (copied). When a microorganism develops a characteristic, such as resistance to an antibiotic, that characteristic is passed to every daughter cell through the DNA. Bacteria obtain antibiotic resistance by mutation (i.e., changes in the sequence of DNA). There are at least four known methods: random mutation, transformation, transduction, and conjugation. Some random mutations are beneficial to the cell, while others may be lethal. The addition or deletion of a single nucleotide (the building blocks of DNA) may confer resistance to an antibiotic, a trait crucial to bacterial survival. Widespread use of antibiotics may actually promote the development and survival of antibiotic resistant strains of bacteria. Transformation is the transfer of free DNA (probably "leaked" from destroyed bacteria) into another bacterium. The new DNA is incorporated into the host, transforming the host and subsequent daughter cells by displaying new characteristics, such as antibiotic resistance. Transduction is the transfer of DNA from one bacterium to another bacterium by a viral carrier, known as a *phage* (a virus that infects bacteria). When the virus replicates in the host bacterium, some of the host DNA may be incorporated within the viral capsule (the coat surrounding the virus). When the virus infects another bacterium, the previous host DNA may then be combined with the new host DNA, providing a trait such as antibiotic resistance. Conjugation, or mating, is another means of transmitting antibiotic resistance. Some types of bacteria possess the ability to join and thus share DNA. Microorganisms have become adept at changing to survive. As scientists develop agents to kill microbial pathogens, these microorganisms change to resist the antimicrobial agent and pass the trait to the next generation. Antimicrobial resistance is one of the most challenging pharmacologic problems in medicine today.

For example, some bacteria produce an enzyme known as penicillinase. This enzyme breaks down penicillin, thus making the drug ineffective (Fig. 5–3). Penicillinase is produced by two common strains of staphylococci. Thus these microorganisms have become resistant to treatment with penicillin. When this happens, new forms of the antibiotic may be developed. For example, methicillin which is not broken down by penicillinase, remains useful for some strains. However, one strain of *Staphylococcus aureus* has now become resistant to methicillin. This strain is known as **methicillin-resistant *Staphylococcus aureus* (MRSA)**. This resistant strain of bacteria is difficult to treat with available agents.

Other pathogens are becoming resistant to more than one antibiotic. For example, multiple antibiotic resistance is found in a strain of the tubercle bacillus (TB), the pathogen that causes tuberculosis. This strain of TB resists several powerful antibiotics, including streptomycin and rifampicin. Similarly, one group of enteric (digestive-tract) bacteria have developed resistance to vancomycin. These bacteria are known as **vancomycin-resistant enterococci (VRE)**. Additional strains of antimicrobial-resistant pathogenic microorganisms will probably be identified in the near future.

The development of resistant pathogens has been linked to the widespread practice of prescribing antibiotics for such nontreatable viral infections as colds. When normal host bacteria are frequently exposed to antibiotics, they have many opportunities to develop resistance; this means an antibiotic may be ineffective against a subsequent bacterial infection because the resistant trait has pervaded the host's bacterial population. Similarly, when patients do not take

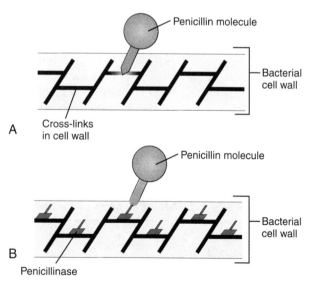

Figure 5–3 Penicillinase inactivates penicillin. (**A**) Penicillin breaks down crosslinks in bacterial cell wall. (**B**) Penicillinase breaks down a portion of penicillin structure, inactivating it.

necessary antibiotics as prescribed—regularly and in the right dose—they give pathogens a chance to develop resistance. Weaker pathogens may be destroyed, but stronger, mutated strains may survive and reproduce.

Antibiotic Agents

Many antibiotics are available to treat a wide variety of infectious processes. In this text, however, we'll focus on the few categories of antibiotics commonly used in surgical procedures (Table 5–3). Antibiotics are usually administered intravenously both before and during a surgical procedure for prophylaxis against surgical wound infections. Antibiotics may also be administered topically, often in the form of irrigant solutions or as ointments. Antibiotics are also prescribed for postoperative use, to be administered intravenously or orally, to prevent or treat infection. Here, we'll look at some common categories of antibiotics, together with their origins, mechanisms, and surgical uses.

Aminoglycosides

Aminoglycosides, which are derived from various strains of *Actinomyces* bacteria, interfere with protein synthesis by binding to bacterial (prokaryotic) ribosomes. They are bactericidal and relatively narrow in spectrum. Generally active only against aerobic, **gram-negative** bacteria, aminoglycosides also provide some activity against some **gram-positive** bacteria such as *Staphylococcus* species, including some methicillin-resistant strains. Otherwise, they are not very active against gram-positive organisms. All aminoglycosides are contraindicated if the patient has a history of hypersensitivity or toxic reactions to any aminoglycoside. Major adverse effects include ototoxicity and nephrotoxicity; i.e., these drugs can damage the auditory nerve and kidney cells. Irreversible deafness, renal failure, and death have been reported after extensive irrigation of surgical fields with aminoglycosides.

Aminoglycosides are poorly absorbed orally, but are almost completely absorbed when applied topically during surgical procedures. Intramuscular and

Table 5–3 Major Groups of Antibiotics

Aminoglycosides
Cephalosporins
Macrolides
Penicillins
Tetracyclines

intravenous injections are the most common administration routes for amino-glycosides.

Aminoglycosides are indicated for short-term treatment of serious infections due to susceptible organisms. Such infections include bacterial septicemia as well as infections of the respiratory tract, bones and joints, central nervous system (meningitis), skin, and soft tissue. They also include intra-abdominal infections.

Among the drugs in the aminoglycoside category are amikacin (Amikin), gentamicin (Garamycin, Jenamicin), streptomycin, tobramycin (Nebcin), neomycin (Neobiotic), and kanamycin (Kantrex), as listed in Table 5–4. Amikacin is often effective even when strains of susceptible organisms are resistant to other amino-glycosides. Gentamicin is available in cream and ointment, ophthalmic solution and ointment, and solution for injection. Streptomycin is used in combination with other agents to treat infections caused by *Mycobacterium tuberculosis* (the tubercle bacillus) and is administered intramuscularly only. Neomycin is too toxic for systemic use, so it is applied topically only.

Cephalosporins

Cephalosporins are broad-spectrum antibiotics derived from the fungus *Cephalosporium acremonium.* Cephalosporins are bactericidal, targeting cell-wall synthesis. That is, they block an enzyme needed to strengthen the bacterial cell wall, causing cell lysis (rupture). We classify cephalosporins into three "generations" based on different ranges of activity:

> *First-generation cephalosporins* are active against many gram-positive and some gram-negative microbes.
> *Second-generation cephalosporins* are effective on a wider variety of gram-negative, but fewer gram-positive organisms.
> *Third-generation cephalosporins* have a wider range of activity against gram-negative microbes than second-generation agents, but are less effective on gram-positive organisms.

Table 5–4   Aminoglycosides

Generic Name	Trade Name
Amikacin	Amikin
Gentamicin	Garamycin, Jenamicin
Streptomycin	
Tobramycin	Nebcin
Neomycin	Neobiotic
Kanamycin	Kantrex

Cephalosporins are used as prophylaxis in a variety of surgical procedures and are often indicated when patients are allergic to penicillins (although some cross-reactivity is possible). Administration is oral, intramuscular, or intravenous, depending on the particular cephalosporin. Table 5–5 lists cephalosporins by generation.

☞ Cephalosporins are among the most expensive antibiotics.

Macrolides

Macrolides, which include the erythromycins, are a group of broad-spectrum agents that inhibit bacterial protein synthesis by binding to the prokaryotic ribosomal subunit. Bacteriostatic for most bacteria, macrolides are bactericidal for several gram-positive bacteria such as *Legionella*. This cidal activity is explained

Table 5–5 Cephalosporins

Generic Name	Trade Name
First-generation	
Cefazolin	Ancef, Kefzol, Zolicef
Cefadroxil	Duricef, Ultracef
Cephalexin	Keflex, Keflet
Cephalothin	Keflin
Cephapirin	Cefadyl
Cephradine	Anspor, Velocef
Second-generation	
Cefoxitin	Mefoxin
Cefaclor	Ceclor
Cefamandole	Mandol
Cefmetazole	Zefazone
Cefonicid	Monocid
Cefotetan	Cefotan
Cefuroxime	Ceftin, Zinacef
Third-generation	
Cefotaxime	Claforan
Cefixime	Suprax
Cefoperazone	Cefobid
Ceftazidime	Ceptaz, Fortaz, Tazicef, Tazidime
Ceftizoxime	Cefizox
Ceftriaxone	Rocephin

by the fact that these antibiotics can penetrate the cell walls of gram-positive organisms. Macrolides may be obtained from isolates of *Streptococcus erythreus* or they may be synthesized in the laboratory. Macrolides are only partially metabolized and are excreted almost unchanged in bile. Most macrolides are administered orally; however, erythromycin is available in topical ointment and solution, as well as in an ophthalmic ointment for local infections. Macrolide antibiotics include erythromycin, erythromycin ethylsuccinate, azithromycin, and clarithromycin, as listed in Table 5–6.

Penicillins

Penicillin was the first of the antibiotics (see Insight 5–3). Originally extracted from the mold *Penicillium,* this antibiotic is now available in many natural and semisynthetic forms effective against a wide variety of gram-positive and gram-negative microbes. Penicillins are bactericidal; they block an enzyme needed to strengthen the bacterial cell wall, so the cell eventually ruptures. Some species of bacteria have become resistant to penicillin by producing *penicillinase,* an enzyme that breaks down the drug molecule. Four basic categories of penicillins are available; natural penicillins, penicillinase-resistant penicillins, aminopenicillins, and broad-spectrum penicillins. Penicillins may be given orally, or by intramuscular or intravenous injection, depending on the agent. Penicillins are often used preoperatively for prophylaxis against surgical wound infections. Allergic reactions to penicillin are common, with cross-reactivity among penicillins and some of the cephalosporins. Table 5–7 lists some of the penicillins by category.

Natural penicillins include penicillin G, penicillin V, and benzathine penicillin G. Advantages of natural penicillins are low cost and low toxicity. Natural penicillins display a relatively narrow spectrum of action, primarily against gram-positive microbes.

Penicillinase-resistant penicillins are semisynthetics that include methicillin, cloxacillin, dicloxacillin, nafcillin, and oxacillin. This class of penicillins was

(Text continues on page 118.)

Table 5–6 Macrolides

Generic Name	Trade Name
Erythromycin	E-mycin, ERYC
Erythromycin ethylsuccinate	EES, Ery Ped
Azithromycin	Zithromax
Clarithromycin	Biaxin

INSIGHT 5-3 ▌ **YESTERDAY AND TODAY: VACCINES AND THE DISCOVERY OF PENICILLIN**

Penicillin, discovered by **Alexander Fleming** in 1928, was the first of the "wonder drugs" known as antibiotics. It revolutionized medicine by fighting bacterial infections—which, at that time, could be deadly complications to any type of wound. A chain of events led to the development of this wonder drug. Prominent in these events were men who would lay the foundations for modern-day bacteriology and immunology.

The first event took place in 1796, more than a hundred years before Fleming's discovery, when **Edward Jenner** discovered a way to prevent smallpox. Jenner was an English country doctor who had observed that dairy maids who contracted a mild infection known as cowpox did not come down with smallpox. So he injected patients with pus from cowpox sores. These injections immunized his patients against smallpox. He knew nothing about the viruses that caused the disease and even less about the antibodies his innoculations stimulated. But his was the first step toward understanding the disease-causing mechanisms of certain microorganisms. The next step was taken in the 1850s when a French chemist named **Louis Pasteur** began work with microscopic organisms called bacteria (or germs). By 1870, he had proved that disease in silkworms was caused by germs. He then reasoned that germs could also cause disease in animals, including humans. But as Pasteur was not a physician, he kept his research centered around animals. Next, he worked with chicken cholera. When he accidentally infected some chickens with an old strain of cholera, he found that the inoculated chickens did not develop the full-blown disease. In fact, the chickens recovered from their mild infection and subsequently proved immune to cholera. Pasteur was familiar with Jenner's work, so he deduced that old or weakened germs could be used to protect people from contracting a particular disease. Pasteur called his inoculum a "vaccine," then went on to develop other vaccines for anthrax and rabies.

Another event took place when a highly respected Scottish surgeon named **Joseph Lister** became interested in Pasteur's work. He reasoned that germs could get into surgical wounds and cause postoperative problems—pus, swelling of tissue, fevers, and (all too often) death. Lister added a surgical link to the chain by using chemicals to kill germs in the operating room. His methods —which included spraying the room with carbolic acid—yielded impressive results. Lister's germ-killing chemicals were the first antiseptics. In the meantime, the chain of events strengthened as a German physician, **Robert Koch,** worked on the role played by bacteria in disease. It was he who proved that specific germs causing diseases in animals caused them in humans as well. In 1876, Koch identified the germ that causes anthrax, showing that it affects cattle, sheep, and people, too. Then, in 1882, he isolated the tuberculosis germ, a common killer of that time.

In 1893, an influential British Army Medical School physician named **Almroth Wright** forged another link in the chain when he began the search for a typhoid vaccine. He was concerned that this disease was a serious threat to soldiers in the field. Spread by unsanitary conditions that contaminated water, milk, or food, typhoid killed 10–30% of its victims at that time. Wright took six years to produce a successful vaccine. Then the army authorities refused to use it on a large scale. As a result, thousands of British troops contracted typhoid during the Boer War (1899–1902), and more troops died of this disease than from battle wounds. Shocked and bitterly chagrined, Wright resigned from the Medical School and joined the faculty at St. Mary's Hospital in London. There he created a department to study germs, immunity, and vaccines. In 1910, Wright hired a new research worker—**Alexander Fleming.**

Fleming and the staff of Wright's "Innoculation Department" took blood and pus samples from patients with ulcers, boils, and sores in order to develop vaccines. They kept their samples in petri dishes filled with agar (a gelatin made from seaweed). Fleming was particularly interested in a pus-producing bacterium called *Staphylococcus,* which is commonly found on the skin. He prepared many microscopic slides from these germ samples. One day, Fleming noticed a mold growing on one of his samples. Molds are simple, nonflowering plants from the fungi family; they can float freely in the air and this one had blown onto his petri dish by accident. But this "spoiled" sample was special: Around the area of the mold was a wide, clean area—no staphylococci. Even beyond this clean area, the staphylococci were dissolving. Clearly, something from the mold was killing the disease-causing germs. Fleming found out the killer mold was a common one, often found on ripened cheese, stale bread, and rotting fruit. It was from the group of molds called *penicillia,* so Fleming named his discovery "penicillin." However, when he announced his discovery to the rest of the department, no one was impressed. Even Wright showed little enthusiasm. Fortunately, Fleming continued his research, growing more of the mold and testing it on a variety of bacteria. Some were not affected, but a number of them were destroyed. Among those affected were the germs that cause pneumonia, scarlet fever, meningitis, diphtheria, and gonorrhea. Then Fleming took the next step. He went on to test the mold on human blood and found it did not kill white blood cells. He successfully used it topically on a lab assistant to cure an eye infection. But Fleming was no chemist, so he had problems extracting and purifying the mold. This left him believing the new medicine was good for topical use only. When he presented a paper on penicillin to a medical audience in 1929, he was met with indifference. Fleming's interest waned and his work was directed along other paths.

Ten years later, a team of Oxford medical researchers picked up where Fleming left off. The Oxford Team took samples of penicillin to the United States, sought backing, and found manufacturers for the new antibiotic. The mass production of this wonder drug in the U.S. was to save millions of Allied soldiers' lives during World War II. And after the War, penicillin and its "wonder-full" derivatives were to change the history of medicine forever.

Table 5–7 Penicillins

Generic Name	Trade Name
Natural penicillins	
Penicillin G	Pentids, Pfizerpen
Benzathine penicillin G	Bicillin L-A, Permapen
Penicillin V	Beepen-VK, Betapen-VK
Penicillinase-resistant penicillins	
Methicillin	Staphcillin
Cloxacillin	Cloxapen
Dicloxacillin	Dycill, Pathocil
Nafcillin	Nafcil, Unipen
Oxacillin	Bactocill
Aminopenicillins (not penicillinase-resistant)	
Ampicillin	Omnipen
Amoxicillin	Amoxil, Polymox
Bacampicillin	Spectrobid
Broad-spectrum penicillins	
Carbenicillin	Geocillin
Mezlocillin	Mezlin
Piperacillin	Pipracil
Ticarcillin	Ticar

developed to be effective against strains of bacteria that produce penicillinase. However, some bacteria have developed a means of resistance against penicillinase-resistant penicillins. MRSA is actually resistant to all penicillinase-resistant penicillins.

Aminopenicillins have been chemically altered by adding an amino group, which makes them effective against gram-negative species, but they are not penicillinase-resistant. These semisynthetics include ampicillin, amoxicillin, and bacampicillin.

Broad-spectrum penicillins include carbenicillin, mezlocillin, piperacillin, and ticarcillin. Broad-spectrum penicillins are semisynthetics that have been chemically altered to be effective against strains of gram-negative microbes.

Tetracyclines

Tetracyclines were the first broad-spectrum antibiotics, originally obtained from cultures of *Streptomyces*. Bacteriostatic action against many gram-positive and gram-negative bacteria, tetracyclines bind to the bacterial ribosomal subunit, interfering with protein synthesis. They also exhibit some action on bacterial cell membranes, causing leakage. Many common bacteria have developed resistance to tetracyclines, so their use is now limited. They are used primarily to treat acne and rickettsial infections.

Tetracycline antibiotics are listed in Table 5–8. Tetracycline hydrochloride is administered orally, as no parenteral form is available. Minocycline may be administered intravenously if the oral route is not feasible. Oxytetracycline may be administered intramuscularly if the oral route is not feasible; it is also available in an ophthalmic ointment combined with polymixin B sulfate. Doxycycline may be administered orally or intravenously. Chlortetracycline hydrochloride is available only in ophthalmic and topical ointment. In septoplasty or tympanoplasty, packing strips may be saturated with chlortetracycline hydrochloride and used as dressings.

Miscellaneous Antibiotics

Many other antibiotics are available for prophylaxis and treatment of infections caused by susceptible microorganisms, as listed in Table 5–9. These include two additional antibiotic categories, several individual agents, and three combination agents.

QUINOLONES

Quinolones are a category of antibiotics that inhibit DNA-gyrase, a protein necessary for bacterial replication. Quinolones have a relatively low toxicity and a broad spectrum of activity against both gram-positive and gram-negative aerobes, including *Pseudomonas.* Quinolones are given orally or intravenously for systemic infections or for urinary tract infections (UTI). Agents include ciprofloxacin, ofloxacin, norfloxacin, and enoxacin.

Table 5–8   **Tetracyclines**

Generic Name	Trade Name
Tetracycline hydrochloride	Achromycin-V, Sumycin
Minocycline	Minocin
Oxytetracycline	Terramycin
Doxycycline	Vibramycin
Chlortetracycline hydrochloride	Aureomycin

Table 5–9 Miscellaneous Antibiotic and Chemotherapeutic Agents

General Categories	Individual Agents	Combination Agents
Quinolones		
Ciprofloxacin (Cipro)	Aztreonam (Azactam)	Coly-mycin S
Ofloxacin (Floxin)	Chloramphenicol (Chloromycetin)	Cortisporin
Norfloxacin (Noroxin)	Clindamycin (Cleocin)	Neosporin
Enoxacin (Penetrex)	Imipenem (Primaxin)	
	Metronidazole (Flagyl)	
	Polymixin B sulfate (Aerosporin)	
	Vancomycin (Vanocin)	
Sulfonamides		
Silver sulfadiazine (Silvadene)		
Sulfisoxazole (Gantrisin)		
Sulfamethoxazole (Gantanol)		
Sulfasalazine (Azulfidine)		
Sulfacetamide sodium (Sodium Sulamyd)		

SULFONAMIDES

Sulfonamides aren't really antibiotics, but they are antimicrobials, more commonly known as sulfa drugs. Sulfonamides are lab-synthesized chemicals that interfere with cell metabolism by inhibiting bacterial synthesis of folic acid. Introduced in 1935 by Gerhard Domagle, sulfonamides are the oldest of the chemotherapeutic agents. They are in limited use today (owing to increasing microbial resistance) but are still prescribed for nonobstructive UTI, severe burns, and superficial eye infections. Sulfonamides are administered orally, topically, and occasionally intravenously. Examples of sulfonamides include silver sulfadiazine, sulfisoxazole, sulfamethoxazole, sulfasalazine, and sulfacetamide sodium. Sulfamethoxazole is also combined with trimethoprim (another antibacterial) and is available as Bactrim and Septra.

INDIVIDUAL AGENTS

Aztreonam (Azactam) is the first drug of a new class of antibacterials called monobactams. Aztreonam is the totally synthetic form of an antibiotic originally isolated from *Chromobacterium violaceum*. It inhibits bacterial cell-wall synthesis, and has a wide spectrum of cidal activity against gram-negative aerobic pathogens. It is available for intramuscular or intravenous injection.

Chloramphenicol (Chloromycetin) is the synthetic form of an antibiotic originally isolated from *Streptomyces venezuelae,* and is structurally different from all other antibiotics. It is bacteriostatic, inhibiting protein synthesis, with a wide range of activity against gram-positive and gram-negative microbes. Chloramphenicol has potential for serious toxicity, so it is used only when less hazardous antibiotics are ineffective. Adverse effects include bone marrow depression and various blood disorders; consequently, chloramphenicol is inappropriate for prophylaxis. Chloramphenicol may be taken orally or injected intravenously; it is also available as a topical ointment, an otic solution, and as an ophthalmic solution and ointment.

Clindamycin (Cleocin) is the synthetic analog of the natural antibiotic lincomycin. It is active against gram-positive and anaerobic bacteria. Used to treat infections in patients who are allergic to penicillin, clindamycin may be administered orally or intravenously. Its high affinity for bone makes it effective in the treatment of osteomyelitis. Additionally, clindamycin may be used to treat serious respiratory, pelvic, and intra-abdominal infections caused by anaerobic bacteria.

Imipenem (Primaxin) has the widest spectrum of activity of all antibiotics currently available. It works by inhibiting bacterial cell-wall synthesis and is available in forms suitable for intramuscular and intravenous administration. Primaxin is indicated only for serious infections, especially polymicrobic infections (caused by several different microbes) and infections caused by bacteria resistant to other antibiotics.

Metronidazole (Flagyl) is a synthetic antibiotic intended for intravenous administration. It is bactericidal against anaerobic gram-positive and gram-negative bacilli. Often used for prophylaxis in colorectal procedures when contamination from enteric anaerobic bacteria is possible, Flagyl is also used to treat postoperative wound infections caused by susceptible anaerobic bacteria.

Polymixin B sulfate (Aerosporin) is a bactericidal antibiotic effective against nearly all species of gram-negative bacilli. It works against bacteria by increasing the permeability of the cell membrane. Polymixin B sulfate is available in powder form, which is reconstituted for topical, intravenous, or intramuscular administration. It is measured in units rather than milligrams.

Vancomycin (Vanocin) is an antibiotic derived from *Amycolatopsis orientalis* used to treat infections caused by MRSA. It is bactericidal, blocking a reaction needed to form crosslinks in the cell wall. Vancomycin also alters cell-membrane permeability and interferes with RNA synthesis. It is administered intravenously and is active against staphylococci, streptococci, and enterococci.

COMBINATION AGENTS

Several antibiotics are combined with other drugs and used to treat specific conditions. Coly-mycin S Otic is a combination drug used topically to treat bacterial infections of the external auditory canal. It is often administered in surgery after myringotomy and insertion of pressure equalization (PE) tubes. Coly-mycin contains two bactericidal antibiotics, colistin and neomycin, in combination with hydrocortisone (a corticosteroid used as an anti-inflammatory agent).

Cortisporin ophthalmic suspension is a drug used topically when an anti-inflammatory agent is needed in combination with an antibiotic. It contains neomycin and polymixin B sulfate with hydrocortisone. Because Cortisporin is in suspension, it must be shaken prior to administration to distribute the drug particles evenly. It is not intended for injection. Cortisporin is also available combined with bacitracin in an ointment.

Neosporin G.U. Irrigant is a combination of neomycin and polymixin B sulfate. It is used as a topical bladder irrigant when the presence of an indwelling urinary catheter increases the risk of bladder infection.

Summary

Antibiotics are antimicrobial agents used in surgery for prophylaxis against wound infections. They are also given to treat postoperative wound infections. Despite meticulous aseptic technique, wound infections may arise when pathogenic microorganisms are transmitted to a susceptible host. When that happens, the causative microbe will be identified, then tested for antibiotic sensitivity before a definitive course of antibiotic therapy can be selected.

Antibiotics work against microbes in five major ways. The agent may inhibit bacterial cell wall synthesis, impede protein synthesis, interfere with nucleic acid (RNA or DNA) synthesis, alter bacterial cell wall function, or disrupt with bacterial cell metabolism. Antibiotics may be bacteriostatic or bactericidal and may have a broad, narrow, or limited spectrum of activity. Some bacteria have developed resistance to some leading antibiotics, making treatment protocols difficult. Antibiotics may be administered orally, intramuscularly, intravenously, or topically, depending on the agent.

Major categories of antibiotics include aminoglycosides, cephalosporins, macrolides (erythromycins), penicillins, and tetracyclines. Several other categories of antibacterials are in use today, as well as several unique agents. Surgical technologists should become familiar with antibiotics used routinely during surgery.

REVIEW

1. What does MRSA stand for? VRE? Why are these important in surgery?
2. Why are antibiotics administered in surgery?
3. Which test is used to identify the organism that causes TB?
4. What does a C&S reveal?
5. Why would a gram stain be ordered during surgery?
6. How do antibiotics work?
7. What is the difference between bactericidal and bacteriostatic?
8. Why is antimicrobial resistance a problem in surgery?

9. How are antibiotics administered in surgery?

10. In what procedures have you scrubbed or circulated when an antibiotic was administered? Which antibiotic was used? What category did the agent belong in? How was it administered?

CHAPTER 6

Diagnostic Agents

Contrast Media
Omnipaque
Hypaque
Dyes
Methylene Blue

Indigo Carmine
Gentian Violet
Staining Agents
Lugol's Solution
Acetic Acid

OBJECTIVES

Upon completion of this chapter you should be able to:

1 List categories of diagnostic agents used in surgery.
2 Give examples of drugs in each category.
3 Discuss the uses of various diagnostic agents in surgery.

KEY TERMS

contrast media Agents used to visualize anatomic structures or abnormalities under radiographic examination.

dye Agent that colors an object; enhances visualization of anatomic structures or abnormalities under direct vision.

Radiopaque Opacity under radiographic examination.
Staining agent Agent that provides visual contrast of tissues.

Pharmacologic agents called **contrast media** are used in certain diagnostic radiographic tests. To perform these tests, a contrast medium is injected into the circulatory system, or instilled into a body cavity; then an x-ray is taken. Many contrast media contain iodine, which is **radiopaque**; the opposite of *radiotransparent*. Thus, for example, anatomic structures that take up iodine appear opaque on radiographic examination; this means that such pathologic conditions as tumors, stones, or blockages become visible. In surgery, these agents are often referred to incorrectly as "dyes."

Dyes are solutions that color or mark tissue for identification. Dyes may be used to mark skin incisions or to enhance visualization of certain anatomic structures during a surgical procedure. Dyes may be applied topically, injected into the bloodstream, or instilled into a body cavity.

Staining agents are used in surgery to help visually identify abnormal cells, most frequently in procedures on the cervix. Staining agents are chemicals in solution that react differently with abnormal cells than with normal cells.

Contrast Media

Contrast media are radiopaque chemicals. Several different contrast media are available for various diagnostic examinations (Table 6–1). Two common contrast media frequently used in surgery will be discussed as examples. The surgical technologist must exercise caution when preparing these agents because they are clear in color and may easily be confused with other clear medications on the sterile back table. All containers and syringes containing contrast media must be clearly labeled to avoid administration errors. Most contrast media are sensitive to light, so they should be stored covered and away from direct lighting. However, these agents may be safely exposed to light when on the sterile back table during a procedure. This is because the duration of exposure is not sufficient to cause damage to the contrast medium.

Most contrast media contain iodine; therefore a thorough patient history of allergies or reactions to iodine must be obtained and noted in the chart. The circulator will also check for a history of patient allergies or reactions to iodine during the preoperative assessment. If the patient has a positive history for iodine reaction, and use of contrast media is anticipated during the surgical procedure, the surgeon should be alerted prior to patient transport to the operating room.

Table 6–1 Contrast Media Used in Surgery

Agent	Purpose
Omnipaque	Intraoperative angiography
Hypaque	Intraoperative cholangiography

Omnipaque

Iohexol (Omnipaque) is a water-soluble iodine-based radiographic contrast medium, containing approximately 45% iodine. Omnipaque is available in various strengths (140, 180, 210, 240, 300, and 350), expressed as milligrams of iodine per milliliter. It comes in glass vials ranging in size from 10 mL to 250 mL. Omnipaque is absorbed from the site of administration into the bloodstream; it undergoes little or no metabolism and is excreted by the kidneys virtually unchanged. It is contraindicated (inappropriate) for use in patients with known hypersensitivity to iodine. Omnipaque may be injected intrathecally or intravascularly, or it may be instilled into a body cavity prior to radiographic examination. Intrathecal (into the lumbar subarachnoid space) injection of Omnipaque is used for myelography and contrast enhancement of computed tomography (CT) myelography to visualize the spinal cord and nerve roots. For many years, myelography was the standard method used to diagnose a ruptured intervertebral disk. Since myelography involves the injection of contrast media and use of x-ray, it is considered an invasive diagnostic examination. In many instances, traditional myelography is being replaced by magnetic resonance imaging (MRI), a noninvasive diagnostic tool.

When injected into a blood vessel, Omnipaque will opacify that blood vessel—and all other vessels in the path of flow—on radiographic examination (angiography). Angiography is used to demonstrate blockages or anatomic abnormalities of the vascular system. Variations of angiography include angiocardiography, aortography, and peripheral arteriography. Angiography may be performed on vessels of the head, neck, abdomen, or kidneys, as well as on peripheral blood vessels. Omnipaque may be used for intraoperative angiography. For instance, it may be used to confirm removal of a blockage in a peripheral vessel, such as after a femoral embolectomy or laser atherectomy.

Excretory urography (Fig. 6–1) may be performed with intravascular injection of Omnipaque. The contrast medium will reach the kidneys in 1–5 minutes, at which time a urogram may be taken to visualize renal structures or detect possible blockage.

Hypaque

Diatrizoate meglumine 60% (Hypaque) is a water-soluble radiopaque contrast medium containing approximately 47% iodine. The percentage given in the name refers to the amount of meglumine per 100 mL of solution, not the amount of iodine. It is supplied in glass vials of 50 mL and 100 mL. Hypaque is NOT intended

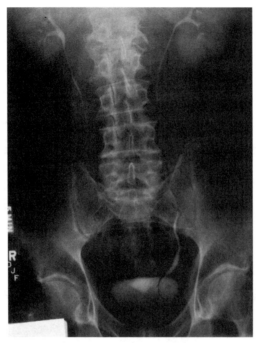

Figure 6–1 Excretory urogram.

for intrathecal administration and is contraindicated in patients with known hypersensitivity to iodine. Common uses for Hypaque include excretory urography, cerebral angiography, peripheral arteriography, and cholangiography.

Hypaque is most frequently used in surgery for operative cholangiograms—open or laparoscopic—to determine the presence of stones in the common bile duct (Fig. 6–2 **A,B**). Often, Hypaque will be diluted at the sterile back table with equal parts of normal saline solution. One method of cholangiography involves attaching one 30-cc syringe filled with saline and one 30-cc syringe filled with Hypaque solution to a three-way stopcock adapter connected to a cholangiogram catheter (Fig. 6–3). Saline is injected into the catheter to verify correct placement; then Hypaque is injected and an x-ray is taken. These syringes must be clearly identified to prevent inadvertent injection of saline prior to radiographic exposure. While saline will not harm the patient, inadvertent injection prior to x-ray will negate the examination and require additional radiographic exposure and extended anesthesia time.

Dyes

Dyes have varied uses in surgery, from marking skin incisions to visual identification of organ injury or pathology. Three of the most common dyes used in surgery (Table 6–2) will be discussed, with examples of practical applications.

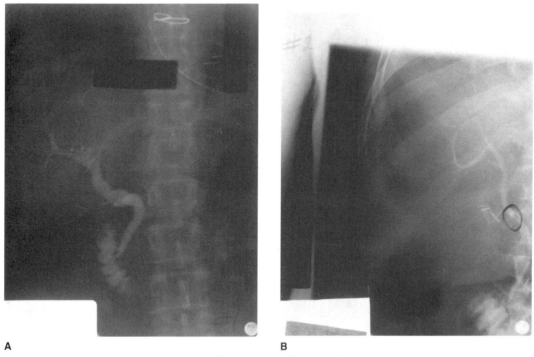

A   B

Figure 6–2 Cholangiogram: (**A**) normal; (**B**) calculus.

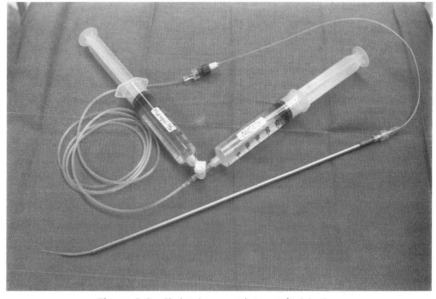

Figure 6–3 Cholangiogram catheter set for injection.

Table 6–2 Dyes Used in Surgery

Agent	Purpose
Methylene blue	Cystoscopy: Detect bladder injury
	Tubal dye studies:Verify patency of uterine tubes
	Bladder surgery or exploration: Detect bladder injury
Indigo carmine	Kidney or bladder procedures: Detect injury to urinary structures
	Verify kidney function during any surgical procedure: Colored urine will be excreted
Gentian violet	Skin marking

Methylene Blue

Methylene blue U.S.P. is available in a 1% solution (10 mg per milliliter of water), packaged in 1-mL and 10-mL vials, or 5-mL ampules. It is most often used in surgery during procedures on the urinary bladder or uterine tubes. Methylene blue is added to a fluid, such as normal saline, to give a deep blue color to the solution. The solution is then instilled into the bladder through an indwelling urinary catheter in order to detect possible injury. If the bladder has a leak or tear, blue solution will be obvious in the pelvis and will be visible as it flows out of the damaged area.

In gynecology, a methylene blue solution is used to demonstrate patency of the uterine tubes. During a procedure called tubal dye study (TDS), or chromotubation, a laparoscope is used to observe the fimbria (ends of the uterine tubes) while methylene blue solution is instilled into the uterus through a special cervical cannula (Fig. 6–4). Methylene blue solution enters the uterine tubes and is observed exiting into the pelvic cavity, verifying patent tubes. If the tubes are blocked, often due to pelvic inflammatory disease, methylene blue solution will not be evident in the pelvis.

Methylene blue may also be used to mark skin incisions. The solution is poured into a medicine cup and a cotton-tipped applicator stick is broken to make a quill-type marker (Fig. 6–5). This marker is dipped into the solution and applied to the skin. In many instances, manufactured skin marking pens are replacing this method.

Indigo Carmine

Indigo carmine is a blue dye that is usually given intravenously to color urine for verification of bladder integrity or kidney function. Each 5-mL of indigo carmine contains 40 mg of indigotindisulfonate sodium in water. It is excreted by the kidneys, usually within 10 minutes after intravenous injection, retaining its color in

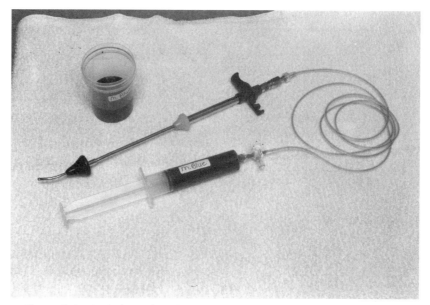

Figure 6–4   Cervical cannula with methylene blue solution for tubal dye study (TDS).

urine. This process allows immediate identification of possible leaks or damage to the ureters or bladder, as well as demonstration of kidney function. Intravenous injection of indigo carmine during cystoscopy may be used to help identify the location of ureteral openings. Indigo carmine is packaged in 5-mL glass ampules and, when stored, should be protected from light.

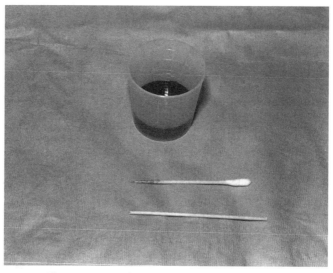

Figure 6–5   Quill-type marker with methylene blue.

Gentian Violet

Gentian violet is a purple dye most frequently used in surgery to mark incision lines. Special sterile marking pens containing gentian violet are available from various manufacturers. These pens are particularly useful for plastic and reconstructive procedures involving complicated incisions such as Z-plasty (Fig. 6–6) or tissue flap grafts. Sterile marking pens may also be used to label containers of medications (Fig. 6–7).

Staining Agents

Staining agents (Table 6–3) may be used in surgery to help identify abnormal tissue for biopsy or excision. Due to differences in cell metabolism between normal and abnormal cells, some chemicals applied to the suspect area react in a way that more clearly demonstrates the location of tissue changes. In surgery, staining techniques are most often used by gynecologists to locate areas of cervical dysplasia for biopsy or excisional conization.

Lugol's Solution

Lugol's solution is a strong iodine mixture used to perform Schiller's test on cervical tissue. For Schiller's test, Lugol's solution is applied topically to the external

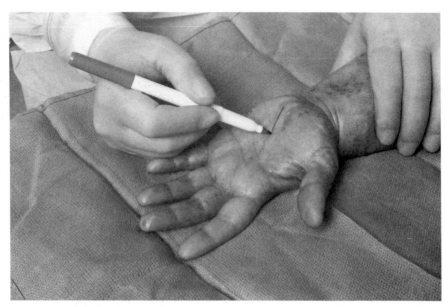

Figure 6–6   Use of a commercial marking pen to mark a skin incision.

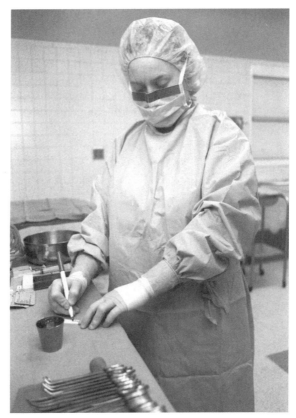

Figure 6–7 Use of a commercial marking pen to label medications.

cervical os with a sponge stick or large cotton-tipped applicator. Abnormal cells will not take up the brown iodine stain as readily as normal cells, visually demonstrating the area of cervical dysplasia to be biopsied. Lugol's solution is contraindicated for use in patients with a history of hypersensitivity to iodine.

Table 6–3 Staining Agents Used in Surgery

Agent	Purpose
Lugol's solution	Schiller's test
Acetic acid	Laser excision of cervical dysplasia

Acetic Acid

Acetic acid (commonly known as vinegar) may also be used to help identify areas of cervical dysplasia. Although it is not specifically a colored staining agent, acetic acid causes abnormal tissue to appear whiter than surrounding healthy tissue. Acetic acid may be used as a staining agent when laser is used to excise dysplasia. Laser energy is absorbed by different colors in the spectrum, and tissue stained brown with an iodine solution may interact less effectively with the laser.

Summary

Several different types of agents are used in surgery to facilitate diagnosis of various pathologic conditions. Diagnostic agents used in surgery fall into three general categories; contrast media, dyes, and staining agents. Contrast media are used to demonstrate anatomic structures or abnormalities under radiographic examination. Dyes color tissue or structures for direct visual examination. Staining agents provide a visual contrast between normal and abnormal tissue.

REVIEW

1. What categories of diagnostic agents are used in surgery?

2. Can you give examples of drugs in each category?

3. How are these diagnostic agents used in surgery?

4. How are categories of diagnostic agents similar? How are they different?

CHAPTER 7

Diuretics

Review of Renal Physiology

Diuretics
High-Ceiling (Loop) Diuretics
Thiazide Diuretics

Potassium-Sparing Diuretics
Carbonic Anhydrase Inhibitors
Osmotic Diuretics

OBJECTIVES

Upon completion of this chapter you should be able to:

1 State the general purpose of a diuretic.
2 Describe the physiology of the kidney.
3 Identify anatomic structures of the nephron.
4 List diseases that use diuretics for management.
5 Describe the impact of long-term diuretic therapy on the patient about to undergo a surgical procedure.
6 Discuss the type of patient who may come to surgery on long-term diuretic therapy.
7 List the two most common diuretics administered intraoperatively and their purpose.

KEY TERMS

Creatinine A nitrogenous compound excreted in the urine.

Electrolyte A chemical substance that dissociates into electrically charged particles when dissolved in water.

Glaucoma A group of diseases of the eye characterized by increased intra-ocular pressure; results in blindness if not treated successfully.

Homeostasis The tendency of biologic systems to maintain relatively constant conditions in the internal environment while continuously interacting with and adjusting to changes originating within or outside the system.

Hyperkalemia Abnormally high potassium concentration in the blood.

Hypokalemia Abnormally low potassium concentration in the blood.

Nephron The structural and functional unit of the kidney.

Diuretics are drugs administered to prevent reabsorption of sodium and water by the kidneys. Diuretics are used in the management of several chronic medical conditions such as congestive heart failure (CHF) and **glaucoma**. Most diuretics also cause excretion of **electrolytes** other than sodium, including potassium and calcium. Potassium (K^+) may be seriously depleted in patients taking certain diuretics, a condition known as **hypokalemia.** If patients on long-term diuretic therapy require surgery, blood chemistry tests will be performed to determine serum potassium levels (normal 3.5–5.0 mEq/L). Potassium levels that are either too low or too high may cause cardiac dysrhythmias under anesthesia (Insight 7–1). Patients with hypokalemia may require administration of intravenous potassium prior to nonemergency surgery. The necessity of preoperative potassium treatment may cause a delay in procedure start time, so operating room staff should be mindful of such possibilities. Long-term diuretic therapy is most frequently seen in elderly patients.

Diuretics are also used during some surgical procedures for short-term reduction of intraocular or intracranial pressure. The risk of hypokalemia is significantly reduced when diuretics are used for treatment of such specific temporary conditions.

In order to understand the action of diuretics, it is necessary to give a brief review of renal physiology. Consult your physiology textbook for additional information.

Review of Renal Physiology

The primary function of the renal (urinary) system is to maintain **homeostasis** by filtering blood and removing excess water and dissolved substances, or *solutes,*

INSIGHT 7–1 | **PHYSIOLOGY INSIGHT: THE IMPORTANCE OF POTASSIUM IN CARDIAC FUNCTION**

Potassium, a mineral element, is the primary intracellular electrolyte in the body. It plays a vital role in many body functions such as nerve impulse conduction, acid–base balance, and promotion of carbohydrate and protein metabolism. Every body cell, especially muscle tissue, requires a high potassium content to function. It facilitates contraction of both skeletal and smooth muscles—including myocardial (heart muscle) contraction. Potassium levels in the body have a very narrow normal range (3.5–5.0 mEq/L) and even a slight deviation in either direction can cause problems. An excess of potassium (*hyper*kalemia) alters the normal polarized state of cardiac muscle fibers. This results in a decrease in the rate and force of the heart's contractions. Very high potassium levels can block conduction of cardiac impulses. This results in rapid heart rate (tachycardia) initially and, later, slow heart rate (bradycardia). If potassium levels are too low (*hypo*kalemia), the heart can develop an abnormal rhythm (arrhythmia). Both hyperkalemia and hypokalemia can lead to muscle weakness and flaccid paralysis. Abnormal potassium levels can diminish excitability and conduction rate of the heart muscle and lead to cardiac arrest. The cause of abnormal levels is usually not dietary deficiency. Many foods contain potassium, including meats, milk, peanut butter, potatoes, bananas, apples, carrots, tomatoes, and dark–green leafy vegetables. Rather, hypokalemia can result from excessive vomiting and diarrhea, severe trauma such as burns, chronic renal disease, excessive doses of cortisone, or thiazide diuretics used to treat hypertension (high blood pressure). Hyperkalemia results from renal dysfunction such as the kidneys' inability to excrete excess amounts of potassium, or when there is decreased urine output or renal failure.

such as sodium and potassium. The **nephron** (Fig. 7–1) is a microscopic filtering unit that removes water and waste solutes. Millions of nephrons are present within the kidneys. Blood is brought to the nephron through the afferent arteriole into Bowman's capsule, where filtration occurs. Filtration is the process of forcing fluids and solutes through a membrane by pressure. Filtered blood then returns to the circulatory system via the efferent arteriole. The remaining fluid, or *filtrate*—which contains all the substances present in blood, except formed elements and most proteins—then undergoes tubular reabsorption. Only specific amounts of needed substances, including water, are reabsorbed. Tubular reabsorption takes place in the proximal convoluted tubule and the ascending and descending limbs of the loop of the nephron (loop of Henle).

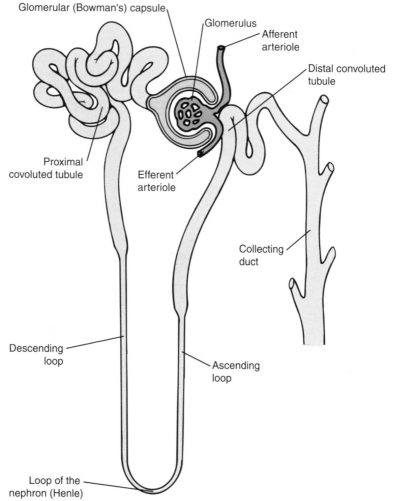

Glomerular (Bowman's) capsule

Glomerulus

Afferent arteriole

Distal convoluted tubule

Proximal covoluted tubule

Efferent arteriole

Collecting duct

Descending loop

Ascending loop

Loop of the nephron (Henle)

Figure 7–1 The nephron.

The filtrate next receives such materials as potassium, **creatinine**, and hydrogen ions from blood surrounding the tubule; this process is called tubular secretion. Tubular secretion, which takes place in the distal convoluted tubule, eliminates waste products and controls blood pH. Additional water is reabsorbed when filtrate proceeds to the collecting ducts. Filtrate is emptied from collecting ducts into the renal pelvis to the ureter and bladder and is excreted as urine.

Diuretics

Most diuretics exert effects at different locations along the nephron. Diuretics cause elimination of excess fluid by preventing reabsorption of sodium and water, increasing urine output. Diuretics are classified by site of action and the mechanism by which the solute is altered (Table 7–1).

Table 7–1 Diuretics by Classification

Class	Generic Name	Trade Name
High-ceiling (loop) diuretics		
	Bumetanide	Bumex
	Ethacrynic acid	Edecrin
	Furosemide	Lasix
Thiazide diuretics		
	Bendroflumethiazide	Naturin
	Chlorothiazide	Diuril
		SK-Clorothiazide
	Hydrochlorothiazide	Esidrix
		HydroDIURIL
		Oretic
Potassium-sparing diuretics		
	Amiloride	Midamor
	Spironolactone	Aldactone
	Triamterene	Dyrenium
Carbonic anhydrase inhibitors		
	Acetazolamide	Diamox
Osmotic diuretics		
	Mannitol	Osmitrol

INSIGHT 7–2 | PATHOLOGY INSIGHT: CONGESTIVE HEART FAILURE

Congestive heart failure, or pump failure, is the inability of the heart to pump sufficient blood to meet the body's demands. Back-pressure from stagnant blood slows down the venous blood return to the heart. When the right ventricle fails, congestion of organs and extremities results. The patient's legs become swollen, especially at the end of the day, and the liver becomes enlarged due to fluid retention. The enlarged liver presses on nerves, which causes pain and nausea. Pressure in the abdominal veins can lead to an accumulation of fluid in the abdominal cavity (ascites). Left ventricular failure leads to pulmonary congestion and edema as fluid builds up in the alveoli. This accumulation of fluids in the lungs causes shortness of breath (dyspnea). As there is less blood flowing to the major organs, their ability to function is impaired. The brain receives less blood, and this means less oxygen (hypoxia). The patient experiences confusion, loss of concentration, and mental fatigue. This also leads to changes in mental status. The kidneys cannot function properly, and this results in less urine formation (oliguria). Renal failure leads to abnormal retention of water and sodium, which leads to generalized edema. Patients with progressive congestive heart failure face life-threatening fluid overload and total heart failure. In order to compensate for decreased cardiac output, the body has adaptive mechanisms to try to meet the body's needs. As the failing heart tries to maintain a normal output of blood, it enlarges the pumping chambers to hold a greater blood volume. This increases the amount of blood pumped with each chamber's contraction. The heart also begins to increase its muscle mass. This allows for more force with each contraction. Along with this, the sympathetic nervous system helps out by activating adaptive processes to increase the heart rate, redistribute peripheral blood flow, and retain urine. These adaptive measures will achieve almost normal cardiac output, but only for a short period of time. They will eventually result in harm to the pump as they require an increase in myocardial oxygen consumption. As the mechanism continues, myocardial reserve is exhausted. This leads to heart failure.

High-Ceiling (Loop) Diuretics

Loop diuretics are used to remove fluid arising from renal, hepatic, or cardiac dysfunction and to treat acute pulmonary edema. Hepatic dysfunction may be due to cirrhosis or liver failure. The most common cardiac dysfunction requiring treatment with diuretics is congestive heart failure (Insight 7–2). The oral form of high-ceiling diuretics may be used in treatment of hypertension. Loop diuretics work by decreasing the reabsorption of Na^+ and Cl^- ions along the whole renal tubule, especially in the loop of Henle. These diuretics exert a potent effect because the site of action is so broad. Examples of loop diuretics are bumetanide (Bumex), ethacrynic acid (Edecrin), and furosemide (Lasix). Furosemide is the most commonly used agent in this category. In surgery, furosemide is particularly useful in intracranial procedures. Furosemide decreases intracranial pressure by quickly removing fluid that accumulates in response to the trauma of intracranial procedures or injuries. When furosemide is administered intravenously, onset of diuresis can be expected within 5–15 minutes and will continue for approximately 2 hours. The initial dose of furosemide is 20–40 mg IV, to be given over a period of 1–2 minutes. A second dose may be administered 2 hours later.

Thiazide Diuretics

Thiazide diuretics are used to treat essential hypertension and mild chronic edema. Thiazides work by inhibiting the reabsorption of sodium (Na^+) and chloride (Cl^-) ions in the ascending loop of the nephron. Examples of thiazide diuretics include bendroflumethiazide (Naturetin), chlorothiazide (Diuril, SK-Clorothiazide), and hydrochlorothiazide (Esidrix, HydroDIURIL, Oretic).

Potassium-Sparing Diuretics

Potassium-sparing diuretics are commonly used to treat edema and hypertension and to help restore potassium levels in hypokalemic patients. Potassium-sparing diuretics are usually administered in combination with other diuretics such as thiazides and loop diuretics to minimize potassium loss. Potassium-sparing diuretics prevent the reabsorption of sodium in the distal tubules by altering membrane permeability. This change in membrane permeability also prevents potassium loss. Potassium-sparing diuretics exert a mild diuretic effect because only a small amount of the glomerular filtrate ever reaches the distal convoluted tubule. Common agents in this category include amiloride (Midamor), spironolactone (Aldactone), and triamterene (Dyrenium). Adverse effects can include **hyperkalemia**.

Carbonic Anhydrase Inhibitors

Carbonic anhydrase inhibitors are used to treat mild acute closed-angle glaucoma and chronic open-angle glaucoma (see Chapter 11). Inhibition of the enzyme carbonic anhydrase results in excretion of large amounts of sodium ions and water. Carbonic anhydrase is active in formation of aqueous humor in the eye. By inhibiting carbonic anhydrase, these drugs decrease production of aqueous humor, thus lowering intraocular pressure. The most common carbonic anhydrase inhibitor is acetazolamide (Diamox). Acetazolamide may be given orally to cataract patients after surgery because pressure may build up in the eye as a response to manipulation of tissues.

Osmotic Diuretics

The mechanism of action of osmotic diuretics is unlike that of any diuretics previously described. Osmotic diuretics actually increase blood pressure and volume by drawing fluid out of tissues and into the circulatory system rapidly. Thus, osmotic diuretics are contraindicated in patients with hypertension and edema. Osmotic diuretics are used to prevent acute renal failure after cardiac surgery, treat increased intracranial pressure, and reduce intraocular pressure. Osmotic diuretics are not used for management of chronic conditions such as congestive heart failure (CHF). As the name implies, these drugs exert their effects through the process of osmosis. Remember, osmosis is the process of water moving through a semipermeable membrane from an area of lesser concentration of solute (e.g., sodium) to an area of greater concentration of solute. Water moves toward the diuretic agent present in the glomerulus, thus preventing it (water) from being reabsorbed. Water is then excreted with the diuretic agent in the urine. There is no significant change in sodium reabsorption, so electrolyte balance should remain relatively unaffected.

The most commonly used osmotic diuretic is mannitol (Osmitrol). Mannitol may be used to provide a rapid reduction in intraocular pressure in patients experiencing acute angle-closure glaucoma. It is administered IV, warmed, through a filter to prevent crystallization. Mannitol may also be given during some neurosurgical procedures to reduce intracranial pressure. In vascular procedures, particularly on the aorta, mannitol may be used to protect kidney function by increasing the volume of fluid entering the kidneys (Fig. 7–2).

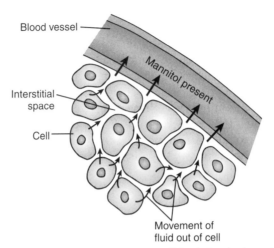

Figure 7–2 Mannitol causes a change in the osmolarity of blood, drawing interstitial and intracellular fluid into the bloodstream. This action eventually increases the amount of fluid excreted by the kidneys.

Summary

Diuretics are agents administered to reduce the amount of fluid accumulating in patients with renal, hepatic, or cardiac dysfunction, as well as to relieve excessive intracranial or intraocular pressure. Excess fluid is removed through excretion of urine. Patients receiving long-term diuretic therapy have an increased risk of hypokalemia. If a surgical patient is hypokalemic, potential exists for cardiac dysrhythmias when under general anesthesia. To detect hypokalemia, blood chemistry analysis is performed preoperatively for all surgical patients taking diuretics.

Some surgical procedures require short-term intraoperative administration of diuretics. Diuretics are given intravenously in surgery during some ophthalmic, intracranial, and vascular procedures. The most common diuretics administered during surgery are mannitol (Osmitrol) and furosemide (Lasix).

REVIEW

1. How does the nephron work to eliminate waste products and excess water?

2. How do diuretics work?

3. Which structures of the nephron are affected by diuretics?

4. Why would a diuretic be prescribed for long-term use?

5. What is a common adverse effect of long-term diuretic therapy on a patient? How does that condition impact the administration of a general anesthetic?

6. What type of patient may come to surgery on long-term diuretic therapy?

7. Why are diuretics used intraoperatively?

8. Which diuretics are used intraoperatively?

CHAPTER **8**

Gastric Drugs

Gastric Physiology Review
Gastric Drug Categories
Antacids
Antiemetics

OBJECTIVES

Upon completion of this chapter you should be able to:

1 Discuss gastric physiology as it affects the surgical patient.
2 List basic categories of gastric drugs.
3 Give an example of each type of gastric drug.
4 Explain the purpose of each gastric drug.

KEY TERMS

Aspiration Inspiration of foreign material into the airway.
Lithiasis A condition marked by formation of calculi and concretions (stones).
NPO Nothing by mouth.

Parietal (oxyntic) cells Acid-secreting cells on the margin of the peptic glands of the stomach.

Peristaltic Pertaining to a wave of contractions passing along a tube.

Prophylaxis Prevention of disease; preventive treatment.

Reflux Backward or return flow.

Regurgitation Backward-flowing process, as in the return of gastric contents into the mouth.

Several types of gastric medications are in current use. Many of these agents are available as over-the-counter (OTC) drugs. Gastric drugs are part of a broader category of drugs that affect the digestive system. Digestive system drugs include laxatives, cathartics, antidiarrheal agents, emetics, antiemetics, and antacids. Of primary concern to the surgical technologist in the clinical setting are gastric drugs, which include antacids and antiemetics. Antacids and antiemetics are administered to the surgical patient preoperatively (see also Chapter 12). A brief review of gastric physiology is presented in order to facilitate understanding of the actions of gastric drugs.

Gastric Physiology Review

The digestive system is responsible for intake and processing of nutrients as well as elimination of nutrient waste. The stomach, which is part of the digestive system, processes food by two means—mechanical and chemical. The mechanical process of digestion is due to the **peristaltic** motions of the muscles and folds (rugae) of the stomach which mix food with gastric secretions. This mixture becomes a thin liquid, called chyme, which is propelled in small amounts through the pylorus into the duodenum. The chemical process of digestion is due to the action of an enzyme called pepsin. In the presence of hydrochloric acid, pepsin becomes active and breaks down protein contained in the ingested food. Hydrochloric acid is produced by the **parietal (oxyntic) cells** of the stomach (see Fig. 8–1) and is the chemical responsible for the acidic nature of gastric contents. Secretion of these chemicals is controlled by both the nervous system and the endocrine system. The nervous system regulates production of gastric chemicals via stimulation of the parasympathetic fibers of the vagus nerve. The sight and smell of food also initiate stimulation of gastric glands to produce digestive chemicals. Ingestion of food then causes stretching of the stomach, which is transmitted through the nerves and a response is generated which produces more stimulation of gastric glands. For further explanation of digestion, consult a physiology textbook.

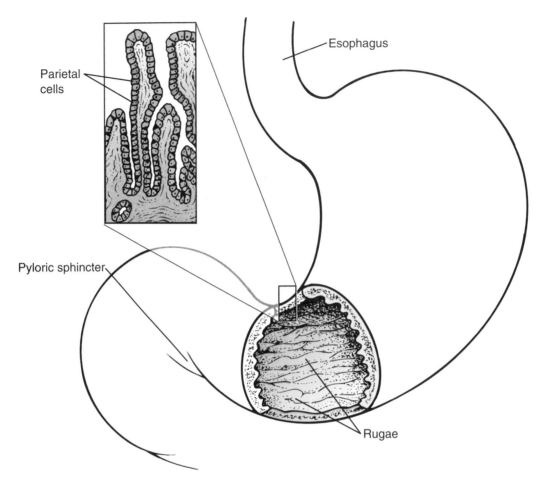

Parietal cells

Esophagus

Pyloric sphincter

Rugae

Figure 8–1 The stomach.

Anxiety and fear, so often seen in surgical patients, initiates a stress response mediated by the sympathetic nervous system which will slow down or stop the digestive process. The presence of food in the stomach and the acidic nature of those contents present a significant hazard to the surgical patient. During induction of general anesthesia, the lower esophageal sphincter and muscles of the thorax may relax to an extent that a **reflux** of gastric contents may occur. In addition, some agents administered at this time may cause nausea, with an increased risk for vomiting. If the patient vomits during induction of anesthesia, gastric contents can enter the lungs, causing severe damage. This potentially fatal complication is called **aspiration**. Elective surgical patients are **NPO**, but gastric secretions are still present. Several agents are used preoperatively to reduce both the risk and potential damage of aspiration (see also Chapter 12).

Gastric Drug Categories

Antacids

PURPOSE

Antacids are drugs that neutralize gastric acid or block production of gastric acid. Antacids are used to treat peptic ulcers, reflux esophagitis, and to prevent stress-induced ulcers and hemorrhage. Antacids such as sodium citrate or histamine (H2) receptor antagonists (blockers) may be ordered preoperatively as **prophylaxis** against aspiration pneumonitis. Oral antacids, such as sodium citrate, are administered preoperatively to neutralize as much gastric acid as possible, reducing potential damage caused if the patient aspirates. Histamine (H2) receptor antagonists are administered to inhibit production of gastric acid. By reducing the amount of gastric acid present, H2 blockers lower potential for lung damage if aspiration occurs. It is important to note that antacids do NOT reduce the possibility of **regurgitation** and aspiration. Antacids are administered to minimize damage that may occur if the anesthetized patient vomits and aspirates gastric contents.

COMMON AGENTS

Medically useful antacids are aluminum hydroxide, calcium carbonate, sodium bicarbonate, and magnesium hydroxide. These chemicals are active ingredients in OTC drugs such as Maalox, Mylanta, and Tums. Common antacids used preoperatively include sodium citrate (Bicitra) and histamine (H2) receptor antagonists (blockers). Cimetidine (Tagamet) and ranitidine (Zantac) are H2 blockers most often used preoperatively. See Table 8–1 for a summary of common antacids.

Table 8–1 Common Antacids Used Preoperatively

Type	Generic Name	Trade Name	Purpose
Oral antacid	Sodium citrate	Bicitra	Neutralize gastric acid (pH)
Histamine (H2) blockers	Cimetidine Ranitidine	Tagamet Zantac	Inhibit production of gastric acid

ACTION

Some antacids such as sodium citrate are chemicals that act as buffers to neutralize hydrochloric acid present in the stomach. In the buffering reaction, gastric acid is neutralized into water and salts. Long-term use of antacids may change urinary pH, causing urinary tract infection (UTI) and possible **lithiasis.** Preoperatively, sodium citrate is administered orally (PO) in doses of 15–30 mL, 15–30 minutes prior to induction of anesthesia. Sodium citrate is intended for short-term use only, so adverse effects are minimized.

Histamine (H2) receptor antagonists work by blocking histamine-induced secretion of hydrochloric acid by gastric parietal cells. The use of H2 blockers significantly reduces the amount of gastric acid present in the stomach. A typical dose of 300 mg of cimetidine is mixed with 50 mL of D5W or normal saline and infused over a period of 15–20 minutes. Ranitidine is usually administered in a dose of 50 mg diluted in 20 mL of normal saline and infused over a period of 5–15 minutes. Histamine (H2) receptor antagonists have no effect on gastric emptying time.

Antiemetics

PURPOSE

Antiemetics are agents that are administered to prevent nausea and vomiting. Some agents are given preoperatively to minimize the possibility of regurgitation and aspiration of gastric contents while under general anesthesia. Other antiemetics may be used postoperatively to prevent nausea and vomiting and thus reduce the potential of surgical wound disruption.

COMMON AGENTS

Several different antiemetics may be used preoperatively (Table 8–2). Drugs that may be administered for their antiemetic effects include droperidol (Inapsine),

Table 8–2 Common Antiemetics Used in Surgery

Generic Name	Trade Name	Purpose
Droperidol	Inapsine	Prevent nausea and vomiting
Metoclopramide	Reglan	Prevent nausea and vomiting; reduce gastric emptying time
Ondansetron	Zofran	Prevent nausea and vomiting

metoclopramide (Reglan), and ondansetron hydrochloride (Zofran). Antiemetics that may be used postoperatively include benzquinamide (Emete-con), diphenidol (Vontrol), and prochlorperazine (Compazine).

ACTION

Nausea and vomiting are responses mediated by an area of the brain in the medulla oblongata (Fig. 8–2) called the chemoreceptor trigger zone. Several antiemetics somehow block receptors in the trigger zone, causing suppression of the nausea/vomiting reflex. The exact mechanism of action of these drugs has not yet been fully explained.

Droperidol (Inapsine) has both sedative and antiemetic properties and is usually administered before surgery intravenously in a dose of 15 µg/kg of patient weight. Onset of the effects of droperidol is expected in 6–10 minutes and will last from 2 to 4 hours.

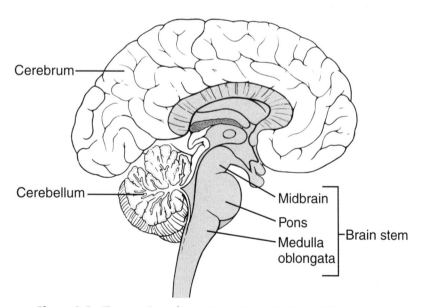

Figure 8–2 The control area for vomiting is located in the medulla oblongata.

Metoclopramide (Reglan) is a gastrointestinal motility agent administered preoperatively for its antiemetic effects. Metoclopramide also stimulates upper gastrointestinal motility and increases lower esophageal sphincter tone. Stimulating upper gastrointestinal motility reduces gastric emptying time, thus reducing the volume of gastric contents. Increasing lower esophageal sphincter tone lowers potential for reflux or regurgitation. Metoclopramide is usually administered intravenously, 10–20 mg over a period of 3–5 minutes, at least 15–30 minutes prior to induction of anesthesia. Onset of effects is seen in 1–3 minutes with a duration of 1–2 hours. Because metoclopramide is a gastric motility agent, it does NOT affect the pH of gastric contents.

Ondansetron (Zofran) was developed to treat nausea in patients undergoing chemotherapy for cancer. It has been found to be an effective antiemetic in surgical patients as well. Ondansetron is usually administered prior to induction of anesthesia intravenously in a dose of 4 mg over a period of 2–5 minutes to prevent postoperative nausea and vomiting.

Summary

Gastric drugs are a subclass of drugs that affect the digestive system. Several gastric drugs are in use today for the treatment and prevention of ulcer disease. In surgery, gastric drugs are used to neutralize or reduce production of gastric acid and to reduce the potential for gastric reflux, vomiting, and aspiration. The gastric drugs used in surgical patients include antacids such as sodium citrate, cimetidine, and ranitidine, as well as antiemetics such as droperidol, metoclopramide, and ondansetron.

R E V I E W

1. How does gastric physiology affect the surgical patient?

2. What are the two basic categories of gastric drugs used in surgery?

3. Can you give an example of each type of gastric drug?

4. What is the purpose of each gastric drug?

CHAPTER **9**

Hormones

Endocrine System Review

Endocrine Glands

Pituitary Gland

Thyroid Gland

Adrenal Glands

Pancreas

Ovaries

Testes

OBJECTIVES

Upon completion of this chapter you should be able to:

1 Define terminology related to the endocrine system.
2 List endocrine glands and hormones secreted by each.
3 State the purpose for administration of each hormone.
4 Match generic and trade names of hormones.
5 Describe surgical uses for hormones.
6 List hormones that may be administered from the sterile field.
7 List procedures that may require administration of hormones from the sterile field.

KEY TERMS

Amenorrhea Absence of the menses.

Androgen Any steroid hormone that promotes male characteristics.

Dysmenorrhea Painful menstruation.

Endometriosis A condition in which tissue resembling endometrium occurs aberrantly in various locations in the pelvic cavity and elsewhere.

Fibrocystic disease of the breast A disorder characterized by single or multiple benign tumors in the breast.

Hyperthyroidism Excessive functional activity of the thyroid gland.

Hypoglycemic drugs Synthetic drugs that lower the blood sugar level.

Hypogonadism Decreased functional activity of the gonads.

Hypothyroidism Deficiency of thyroid gland activity.

Palliative Treatment affording relief but not cure.

Recombinant DNA technology The process of taking a gene from one organism and inserting it into the DNA of another; also called genetic engineering or biotechnology.

Hormones are chemicals released by endocrine glands into the bloodstream (Fig. 9–1). These diverse substances maintain homeostasis by altering the activities of specific target cells. Functions regulated by hormones include reproduction, growth and development, and metabolism. Hormones have a wide range of actions and effects and each hormone has a specific function at a specific location in the body. In addition to naturally occurring hormones, several synthetic hormones have been developed. Most hormones are administered as replacement therapy in the medical rather than the surgical setting. But some hormones are used in surgery and may be administered from the sterile back table during the course of a procedure.

Endocrine System Review

The endocrine system works with the nervous system to relay messages to maintain homeostasis. The endocrine system communicates by sending chemical messengers (hormones) to target cells located all over the body. Hormones are produced by endocrine glands and secreted into the extracellular space. They enter capillaries and are carried by the bloodstream to target cells. Hormones bind to receptor sites on cells and cause a change in cell physiology. Chemical messages take longer to work than those relayed by the nervous system, but effects generally last longer. Hormonal effects are many and varied, but actions on the body may be categorized into four main groups:

- Regulation of internal chemical balance and volume

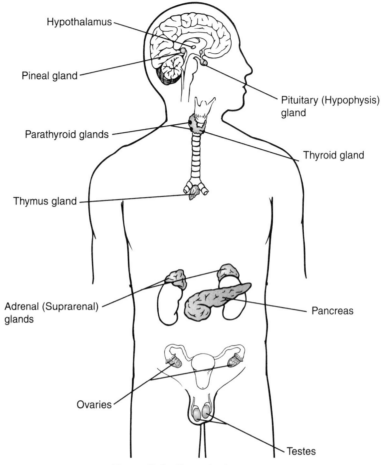

Figure 9–1 The endocrine system.

- Response to environmental changes, including stress, trauma, temperature changes, etc.
- Growth and development
- Reproduction

Hormones may be classified as steroid and nonsteroid. Steroid hormones are derived from cholesterol and include aldosterone, cortisol, estrogen, progesterone, and testosterone. Nonsteroid hormones are synthesized from amino acids. The simplest hormones are amines, derived from a single amino acid. Amine hormones include epinephrine, norepinephrine, thyroxine, and tri-iodothyronine. Hormones made of short chains of amino acids are called peptide hormones. Antidiuretic hormone (ADH) and oxytocin are examples of peptide hormones. Protein hormones are longer, folded chains of amino acids. Examples of protein hormones are growth hormone (GH), parathyroid hormone (PTH), insulin, and glucagon.

The vast majority of endocrine disorders are due either to hyposecretion or hypersecretion of hormones. Treatment for hyposecretion may include administration of hormones to supplement or replace hormones. Hypersecretion may be treated medically with drugs to reduce secretion or surgically by gland removal, depending on indications.

Endocrine Glands

Pituitary Gland

The pituitary gland, known as the "master gland," has a vital role in reproduction and growth, while it regulates the function of the renal system and thyroid gland. The pituitary gland is divided into two lobes—the adenohypophysis and the neurohypophysis. Hormones secreted by the adenohypophysis include growth hormone (GH), thyroid-stimulating hormone (TSH), adrenocorticotropic hormone (ACTH), and gonadotropic hormones. The neurohypophysis secretes oxytocin and antidiuretic hormone (ADH).

It is now possible to synthesize human growth hormone by **recombinant DNA technology**. It is used for long-term treatment of children with growth failure due to hyposecretion of GH.

A pituitary hormone of particular importance to the surgical technologist is oxytocin. Oxytocin stimulates the uterine contractions necessary for normal labor and delivery. If a patient is unable to produce sufficient oxytocin naturally, it may be administered intravenously to induce labor. After delivery of the infant, the uterus must continue to contract in order to expel the placenta and to stop postpartum bleeding from the placental attachment site. After a cesarean section, the uterus will be examined for sufficient contractions to naturally stop postpartum bleeding. If natural contractions are not firm enough, oxytocin may be injected directly into the uterine muscle. The scrubbed surgical technologist will use a syringe to draw up the desired dose of oxytocin from a vial held by the circulator, change needles, then pass the medication to the surgeon. Oxytocin is available as Oxytocin, Pitocin, and Syntocinon.

☞ It is critical to avoid confusion of Pitocin with Pitressin. Pitocin is oxytocin, but Pitressin is vasopressin, which contains antidiuretic hormone (ADH) and oxytocin in a ratio of 20:1. It is used subcutaneously or intramuscularly to stabilize fluid balance in patients with diabetes insipidus. The surgical technologist must be alert to drug names that sound similar. When in doubt, always clarify the order.

Thyroid Gland

The thyroid gland is a vascular structure consisting of two lobes joined by an isthmus. The largest of the endocrine glands, the thyroid is located below the larynx, on both sides of the trachea in the anterior neck. It sets the rate of body metabolism. In children an underfunctioning thyroid (**hypothyroidism**) can stunt growth and retard mental development. Lack of thyroid hormones slows metabolism. An adult with **hypothyroidism** is sleepy, tires easily, is less mentally alert, has reduced endurance, and has a slow heart rate (bradycardia). Overfunctioning of the thyroid, called Grave's disease or hyperthyroidism, causes restlessness, nervousness, sweating, and tachycardia (rapid heart rate). The thyroid secretes three important hormones: thyroxine, triiodothyronine, and calcitonin. Thyroxine (T4) and triiodothyronine (T3) are regulated by thyroid-stimulating hormone (TSH), which is produced in the pituitary gland. These hormones are essential for normal growth and development; they also help regulate metabolism of carbohydrates, lipids, and proteins. Both T3 and T4 require iodine salts for production. Iodine salts are obtained from foods after absorption through the intestines. After absorption, iodine salts are transported by the bloodstream to the thyroid for use in hormone production. Calcitonin helps to control calcium and phosphate concentrations in the blood, and it is regulated by blood levels of these ions. Calcitonin can affect calcium and phosphate levels by inhibiting the rate of release from bone, increasing the rate of incorporation of these ions into bone, and increasing excretion of these ions by the kidneys.

Thyroid hormones are administered to treat hypothyroidism caused by disease or surgical removal of the thyroid gland. Naturally occurring thyroid hormone has been extracted from the thyroid gland of pigs (porcine) and is labeled as desiccated thyroid (Thyroid USP) and thyroglobulin (Proloid). Many types of synthetic thyroid hormone are available, including levothyroxine (Levothroid, Synthroid), liothyronine (Cytomel), and liotrix (Euthroid, Thyrolar). See Table 9–1 for a summary of thyroid hormones.

Antithyroid hormones may be used to treat hyperthyroidism. A common antithyroid agent is methimazole (Tapazole), which may be used before surgery to reduce the size of a thyroid tumor or to inactivate thyroid tissue.

Table 9–1   Thyroid Hormones

Generic Name	Trade Name
Desiccated thyroid	Thyroid USP
Thyroglobulin	Proloid
Levothyroxine	Levothroid
	Synthroid
Liothyronine	Cytomel
Liotrix	Euthroid
	Thyrolar

Adrenal Glands

The adrenal glands are pyramid-shaped glands positioned on top of each kidney. The adrenals are very vascular and consist of a central portion, the medulla, and an outer portion, the cortex. The adrenal medulla produces, stores, and secretes the hormones epinephrine (adrenalin) and norepinephrine (noradrenalin), collectively called catecholamines. The catecholamines are *sympathomimetic,* meaning they mimic effects of the sympathetic portion of the autonomic nervous system. Epinephrine and norepinephrine work with the sympathetic nervous system to prepare the body for the "fight-or-flight" response to stress. Effects of these hormones include increased heart rate, increased force of cardiac muscle contraction, vasoconstriction, elevated blood pressure, increased respiratory rate, and decreased digestive system activity.

Epinephrine is of particular interest to the surgical technologist because it is used frequently in surgery. Epinephrine is often used in combination with local anesthetics to prolong anesthesia. When injected in dilute amounts (1:100,000 or 1:200,000), epinephrine causes local vasoconstriction; this means it reduces blood flow so it reduces the absorption rate of the anesthetic. Epinephrine may also be used topically for hemostasis. In middle ear procedures, for example, tiny pledglets of Gelfoam are typically dipped in more concentrated epinephrine (1:1000) and applied to areas of capillary bleeding. Epinephrine 1:1000 is always used for topical application—never injection. If epinephrine 1:1000 is injected, deadly tachycardia and hypertension may result. Often, a local anesthetic will be combined with dilute epinephrine, then injected to help control bleeding in middle ear procedures. As an example, in tympanoplasty, epinephrine in two strengths may be on the back table (1:1000 for topical only; 1:100,000 or 1:200,000 in local anesthetic for injection). Both solutions are clear. The scrubbed surgical technologist *must* know the route for each administration strength of epinephrine in order to pass each at the correct time. The scrub must carefully label each drug—its identity *and* its strength—as it is accepted into the sterile field to avoid errors.

Adrenal cortex hormones are classified in two major groups—glucocorticoids and mineralocorticoids—collectively known as steroids. The most important mineralocorticoid is aldosterone, which maintains homeostatic levels of sodium in the blood. Most significant to the surgical technologist are the glucocorticoids, which are used to reduce or inhibit the inflammatory response after surgical procedures such as shoulder arthroscopy or cataract extraction. Steroids are used medically to help prevent rejection of donated organs, to reduce the inflammatory response in patients with arthritis, and as replacement therapy for Addison's disease (see Insight 9–1). Steroids administered for diseases such as arthritis are used as **palliatives.** Palliative drugs relieve symptoms, but they do not cure the condition.

Steroids may be administered orally, topically, intramuscularly, or rarely, intravenously. Hormones may be long- or short acting, depending on the agent used. Naturally occurring steroids include cortisone, hydrocortisone, aldosterone, and deoxycorticosterone. Many synthetic steroids have been produced.

INSIGHT 9–1 | **PATHOLOGY INSIGHT: ADDISON'S DISEASE**

Addison's disease, also known as adrenocortical hypofunction, occurs when the adrenal cortex does not secrete adequate amounts of steroid hormone. The disorder was first described by Thomas Addison in 1855, when the primary cause was tuberculosis. Today, however, autoimmune disease is the most common cause. Why? Because the body's circulating antibodies react specifically against adrenal tissue to destroy it. Tumors or hemorrhage of the adrenal glands can also cause the disorder, as can hypopituitarism (decreasing adrenocorticotropic hormone [ACTH] secretion) or abrupt withdrawal of long-term corticosteroid treatment. The disorder can occur at any age, even infancy, and is found in both males and females. Medical treatment involves replacement hormones such as prednisone or hydrocortisone drugs and fludrocortisone. John F. Kennedy suffered from Addison's disease. He had almost no adrenal tissue; but by taking replacement hormones, he was able to function in one of the world's most demanding jobs — the presidency of the United States (1960–1963).

A partial list of synthetic steroids includes synthetic cortisone (Cortisone, Cortone), synthetic hydrocortisone (Hydrocortone, Cortef, Solu-cortef), prednisone (Deltasone, Deltra), prednisolone (Delta-cortef, Hydeltra TBA), methylprednisolone (Medrol, Depo-medrol, Solu-medrol), triamcinolone acetonide (Aristocort, Kenacort, Kenalog 40), dexamethasone (Decadron), and betamethasone (Celestone). See Table 9–2 for a summary of generic and trade names of glucocorticoids.

Pancreas

The pancreas, which is posterior to the stomach and behind the parietal peritoneum, is divided into three anatomic areas: the head, which lies within the loop of the duodenum; the body, and the tail. A unique feature of the pancreas is that it functions as an exocrine gland for digestion and as an endocrine gland for release of hormones. The exocrine pancreas is the primary source for the vital digestive enzymes amylase, lipase, and proteinase. A duct from the gland—the pancreatic duct—transports these digestive enzymes to the duodenum.

The endocrine portion of the pancreas is closely associated with blood vessels, which facilitate the transport of pancreatic hormones to the body. Pancreatic hormones are produced by clusters of cells called the islets of Langerhans. Two pancreatic hormones, insulin and glucagon, regulate metabolism of glucose, a simple sugar used as an energy source. Glucagon is a protein; it stimulates the liver to break down glycogen into glucose, thus increasing blood sugar levels. Insulin, also a protein, stimulates the liver to form glycogen from glucose, thus lowering blood sugar levels. In patients with type I diabetes, the body fails to

Table 9–2 Common Glucocorticoids

Generic Name	Trade Name
Cortisone	Cortisone
	Cortone
Hydrocortisone	Hydrocortone
	Cortef
	Solu-cortef
Prednisone	Deltasone
	Deltra
Prednisolone	Delta-cortef
	Hydeltra TBA
Methylprednisolone	Medrol
	Depo-medrol
	Solu-medrol
Triamcinolone	Aristocort
	Kenacort
	Kenalog 40
Dexamethasone	Decadron
Betamethasone	Celestone

produce insulin, so an outside source must be provided. Insulin was first obtained from animals, but human insulin (Humulin) is now produced via recombinant DNA technology.

In type II diabetes, the body fails to respond to the action of insulin on target cells. Type II diabetes may be effectively managed with diet and exercise and/or administration of oral **hypoglycemic drugs,** which include glyburide (Diabeta), chlorpropamide (Diabinese), and tolazamide (Tolinase).

Ovaries

The ovaries, located in the pelvic area, are paired glands that produce estrogen and progesterone. Estrogen and progesterone critical to the development and maintenance of female sex characteristics, including the menstrual cycle, pregnancy, and lactation. These hormones are available in several forms—tablets, capsules, and oil (IM use only)—and are administered to treat **amenorrhea, dysmenorrhea,** and the side effects of menopause. Estrogen and progesterone are used as replacement therapy after menopause or oophorectomy to prevent osteoporosis (see Insight 9–2) and as oral contraceptives. Estrogens are also used for palliative treatment of advanced androgen-dependent prostate cancer and metastatic breast cancer. Common estrogens available are chlorotrianisene (TACE), conjugated estrogens (Premarin), and estradiol (Estrace). Estrogen, which is also available in creme form, is occasionally used on vaginal packing placed after vaginal hysterectomy. One type of progesterone available is medroxy-progesterone (Provera).

INSIGHT 9-2 | **PATHOLOGY INSIGHT: THE ROLE OF ESTROGEN IN OSTEOPOROSIS**

Osteoporosis is a disorder in which the skeletal system loses too much mineralized bone volume. Normal bones are remodeled throughout life. Until about age 30, bone formation exceeds bone resorption. Later, however, bone resorption outpaces formation; the result is a net bone loss of about 0.5% per year after age 30. After menopause, bone resorption is accelerated in women because estrogen production decreases. Bone tissue needs estrogen in order to absorb calcium. Estrogen also increases vitamin D metabolism — a process necessary for calcium absorption from the intestines. Without proper levels of estrogen in the body, the amount of calcium stored in bones is diminished and bones become more porous—i.e., osteoporotic. The skeleton weakens so it is less able to support body weight. Osteoporotic bone can be seen on routine spine x-rays. The shape of the bone is the same, but the image is less distinct; this suggests porous, or weaker, bone. A more sensitive test is a bone-density scan known as dual x-ray absorptiometry, or DEXA. Many times, however, the first indication of osteoporosis is a fracture—in the femur at the hip, in the radius near the wrist, or as compression fractures of the vertebrae. Over time, osteoporotic symptoms include loss of height, stooped posture, and back pain. Estrogen replacement plays an important role in the treatment plan for osteoporosis. In addition, patients receive dietary calcium or calcium supplements together with a regular, reasonable exercise regimen.

Testes

The testes are paired glands located in the scrotum. Endocrine cells are distributed throughout the testes and produce male sex hormones called **androgens.** Androgens, primarily testosterone, are critical for the development of male sex organs and maintenance of secondary sex characteristics. Androgens, especially testosterone (Depo-Testosterone, Delatest), are administered if replacement therapy is indicated, as seen in **hypogonadism.** Testosterone may also be used to treat some types of advanced breast cancer in females. The androgen danazol (Danocrine) is used to treat diseases in females such as **endometriosis** and **fibrocystic disease** of the breast. Patients scheduled for an endometrial ablation may be placed on Danocrine therapy a few weeks prior to surgery to reduce the volume of the endometrial layer.

Summary

Hormones are chemical substances secreted by endocrine glands. Hormones function to maintain the natural equilibrium of the body. As chemical messengers, hormones produce a vast array of effects and act on virtually every cell of the body. Most hormones are administered in the medical setting to replace inadequate amounts of naturally occurring substances. The hormones most commonly administered in surgery are oxytocin, epinephrine, and steroids.

REVIEW

1. What is the purpose of the endocrine system?

2. Why are the following hormones administered?
   thyroid   insulin
   cortisone   estrogen
   testosterone   oxytocin

3. Match the generic drug with the trade name.

   _____ methimazole   **a.** Celestone
   _____ levothyroxine   **b.** Cortone
   _____ dexamethasone   **c.** Danocrine
   _____ betamethasone   **d.** Decadron
   _____ cortisone   **e.** Levothroid
   _____ oxytocin   **f.** Pitocin
   _____ danazol   **g.** Pitressin
   _____ vasopressin   **h.** Tapazole

4. Why would a male receive a female hormone? Why would a female receive a male hormone?

5. What is the purpose of Pitocin? Pitressin?

6. Which surgical procedures may involve the administration of hormones? Which hormones? How will they be administered?

CHAPTER **10**

Drugs That Affect Coagulation

Physiology of Clot Formation

Coagulants
Hemostatics
Systemic Coagulants

Anticoagulants
Parenteral Anticoagulants
Oral Anticoagulants
Thrombolytics

OBJECTIVES

Upon completion of this chapter you should be able to:

1 Define terms related to blood coagulation and drugs that affect coagulation.
2 Describe the physiology of blood clot formation.
3 List agents that affect coagulation by category.
4 Describe the action of drugs that affect coagulation.
5 List uses, route(s) of administration, side effects, and contraindications for drugs that affect coagulation.
6 Describe the impact of preoperative oral anticoagulant therapy on the surgical patient.
7 List examples of surgical procedures in which agents that affect coagulation are administered.
8 Compare and contrast administration route, onset of action, antagonist, and purpose of parenteral and oral anticoagulants.

KEY TERMS

Anticoagulants Agents that inhibit blood clotting.

Coagulation (clotting) factors A series of twelve factors essential to normal blood clotting.

Coagulants Agents that promote, accelerate, or make possible blood coagulation.

Hemostatics Agents that enhance clot formation and reduce bleeding.

Parenteral Administration route other than the alimentary canal (e.g., intramuscular, intravenous, subcutaneous).

Platelet aggregation Clumping together of platelets; part of a sequential mechanism leading to blood clot (thrombus) formation.

Systemic Pertaining to or affecting the body as a whole.

Thrombolytics (fibrinolytics) Agents that dissolve blood clots.

Thrombosis Abnormal formation or presence of a blood clot within a blood vessel.

Blood naturally contains both **coagulants** and **anticoagulants,** which promote and inhibit clotting. Normally, anticoagulants are dominant; they keep blood in liquid form. But when damage occurs to blood vessels, the body's coagulation mechanism begins clot formation to prevent excessive blood loss. At times, it becomes necessary to enhance or assist natural coagulation. During surgical intervention, the blood supply to an area may be disrupted, causing blood loss. While damaged large blood vessels are controlled with electrocautery or ligatures, the natural coagulation process usually works effectively on capillaries, arterioles, and venules. But this process may be assisted. Topical **hemostatics** are coagulants used on areas of capillary bleeding as an adjunct to natural hemostasis. And when natural **coagulation factors** are absent or insufficient, **systemic** coagulants are used to restore or enhance the coagulation process. Although systemic coagulants are usually administered in the medical setting, they may be given immediately preoperatively or intraoperatively.

Conversely, blood coagulation may also be undesirable. Systemic anticoagulants are used to prevent or delay the onset of the coagulation sequence during surgical procedures performed on blood vessels, for example. Heparin is such a systemic anticoagulant. It is routinely administered during peripheral and cardiovascular surgical procedures to prevent adverse clotting. Most other systemic anticoagulants are administered in the medical setting to prevent conditions such as deep vein thrombosis (DVT) or pulmonary embolism (PE). Patients on long-term anticoagulation require special consideration when undergoing an invasive surgical procedure due to delayed coagulation time.

When a blood clot, or thrombus, forms, a mechanism in the blood acts to dissolve the clot naturally. If the natural anticoagulation process is inadequate, **thrombolytics** may be administered to speed clot breakdown. Thrombolytics are used to treat DVT, PE, coronary artery thrombosis, and myocardial infarction.

Physiology of Clot Formation

The body's coagulation mechanism prevents blood loss due to trauma or damage to small blood vessels. (Trauma to large blood vessels, however, requires surgical intervention—electrocautery or ligatures—to control blood loss.) Damage to a small blood vessel causes spasm, which causes a platelet plug to form, which leads to coagulation. In fact, blood clot formation is a cascade of events occurring in three basic stages (Fig. 10–1).

Stage 1: Thromboplastin (also known as prothrombin activator) is formed.
Stage 2: Thromboplastin converts prothrombin (known as factor II) into thrombin.
Stage 3: Thrombin converts fibrinogen (known as factor I) to fibrin.

Fibrin is a mesh of protein threads—a "net" that traps blood cells to form a clot.

Stage 1 involves two different mechanisms for the formation of thromboplastin—the extrinsic pathway and the intrinsic pathway. The *extrinsic* pathway is initiated by factors outside the blood. It is triggered by a clotting factor released from damaged tissue, i.e., tissue thromboplastin, or factor III. The extrinsic pathway can produce a clot in seconds. Tissue thromboplastin (factor III) combines with antihemophilic factor VIII [AHF] and calcium to activate the Stuart-Prower factor X. When activated, factor X reacts with proaccelerin (factor V) and calcium to form thromboplastin.

The *intrinsic* pathway is initiated by substances contained in the blood. This pathway is more complex, and takes several minutes. When a blood vessel is dam-

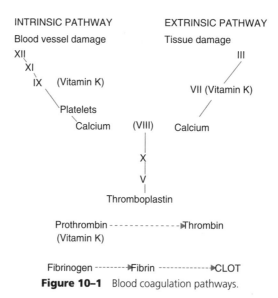

Figure 10–1 Blood coagulation pathways.

aged, the Hageman factor (factor XII) is activated. Factor XII then activates plasma thromboplastin antecedent (PTA; factor XI), which activates plasma thromboplastin component (PTC; factor IX). Then, as in the extrinsic pathway, activated factor IX combines with antihemophilic factor and calcium to activate factor X and factor X reacts with proaccelerin (factor V) and calcium to form thromboplastin.

The clotting cascade requires calcium at all stages—that is, calcium enables many of the steps. Vitamin K also plays a vital role in coagulation. It is required, for example, to synthesize prothrombin (factor II), proconvertin (factor VII), plasma thromboplastin component (factor IX), and the Stuart-Prower factor (X). See Table 10–1 for a summary of blood coagulation factors.

Occasionally, clotting may take place within an unbroken blood vessel; this abnormal clotting is called **thrombosis.** If it forms in an artery, such a clot (thrombus) may cut off blood supply to an area. If a thrombus forms in a vein, it may inhibit return of blood to systemic circulation. Or a clot may break off and become an embolus—traveling to the heart, brain, or lungs—causing severe complications, even death. Blood clots may dissolve naturally; this is because blood normally contains a clot-dissolving enzyme, fibrinolysin. But if the body's natural declotting mechanism is inadequate, medical or surgical intervention may be required. For example, arterial embolectomy may be necessary when blood clots form in the femoral artery. But if a blood clot forms in a vein, medical treatment may be sufficient. With bed rest and administration of thrombolytic agents, such a clot may dissolve.

Table 10–1 Blood Coagulation Factors

Factor	Name	Function
I	Fibrinogen	Converted to fibrin
II	Prothrombin	Converted to thrombin
III	Tissue thromboplastin	Triggers extrinsic pathway
IV	Calcium	Essential in all three stages of clotting
V	Proaccelerin	Accelerates conversion of prothrombin to thrombin
VI		Factor VI is no longer believed to be involved in blood coagulation.
VII	Proconvertin	Essential for extrinsic pathway
VIII	Antihemophilic factor	Accelerates activation of factor X
IX	Plasma thromboplastin component (Christmas factor)	Essential for intrinsic pathway; accelerates activation of factor X
X	Stuart-Prower factor	Essential for intrinsic and extrinsic pathways
XI	Plasma thromboplastin antecedent	Essential for intrinsic pathway; accelerates activation of factor IX
XII	Hageman factor	Essential for intrinsic pathway
XIII	Fibrin-stabilizing factor	Strengthens fibrin clot

Coagulants

Coagulants are drugs that promote, accelerate, or make possible blood coagulation. There are two major categories of coagulants: hemostatics and systemic coagulants. Hemostatics are topical agents used almost exclusively in the surgical setting. Systemic coagulants are generally used in the medical setting.

Hemostatics

Hemostatics are agents that enhance or accelerate blood clotting at a surgical site. These agents serve as adjuncts to natural coagulation, which controls minor capillary bleeding. Thus, hemostatics are not effective against arterial or major venous bleeding. Hemostatics used in surgery are applied topically in the form of films, powders, sponges, or solutions. Several different types of hemostatic agents are available (Table 10–2), and each is supplied in sterile packaging for delivery to the sterile field.

Table 10–2 Topical Hemostatics by Category

Absorbable gelatin
  Gelfilm
  Gelfoam powder
  Gelfoam sponge

Microfibrillar collagen hemostat
  Avitene
  Instat MCH

Oxidized cellulose
  Oxycel
  Surgicel
  Surgicel NuKnit

Absorbable collagen sponge
  Collastat
  Helistat
  Hemopad
  Instat
  Superstat

Thrombin
  Thrombogen

Bone wax

Chemical hemostatics
  Tannic acid
  Silver nitrate

ABSORBABLE GELATIN

Absorbable gelatin hemostatics are animal in origin, made from purified pork skin gelatin USP. Applied topically, with pressure, to bleeding sites, these agents are thought to be mechanical, rather than chemical, in their mode of action. Gelatin hemostatics are absorbed completely in four to six weeks, depending on such factors as the amount used and the surgical site. Gelatin hemostatics may be used dry or moistened with saline; however, they should not be used in the presence of infection or in combination with thrombin. (Such combined use has not been evaluated in controlled clinical trials; thus, it is not recommended by the manufacturer.) Examples of gelatin hemostatics include Gelfilm as well as Gelfoam powder and sponges (Fig. 10–2). Dry Gelfilm has the consistency of stiff cellophane; moistened, it becomes pliable. As a film, it can be cut into desired shapes and sizes. Gelfilm may be used, for example, to pack the area around a tympanic graft. Gelfoam powder can be made into a paste by mixing with saline. The powder form promotes granulation tissue, so it may be used on areas of skin ulceration. Gelfoam sponges are also available. They come in many sizes (Table 10–3) for various applications, and may be torn or cut to desired shapes. Gelfoam is commonly used in orthopedic, general, and neurosurgical procedures.

MICROFIBRILLAR COLLAGEN HEMOSTAT

Avitene is a dry, fibrous preparation of purified bovine corium collagen. Direct application to bleeding surfaces attracts platelets to the substance, thus trig-

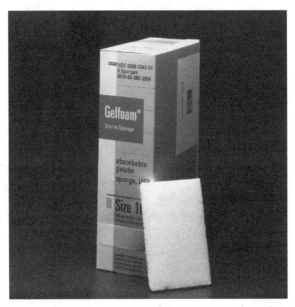

Figure 10–2 Gelfoam. (Photo courtesy of Pharmacia & Upjohn, Kalamazoo, MI.)

Table 10–3 Gelfoam Sponge Sizes

Manufacturer's Code	Actual Size
12-3	20 mm × 60 mm (12 sq cm) × 3 mm thick
12-7	20 mm × 60 mm (12 sq cm) × 7 mm thick
50	80 mm × 62.5 mm (50 sq cm) × 10 mm thick
100	80 mm × 125 mm (100 sq cm) × 100 mm thick
200	80 mm × 250 mm (200 sq cm) × 10 mm thick

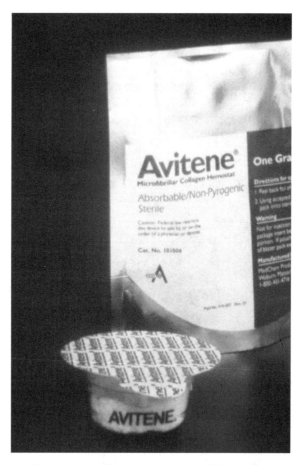

Figure 10–3   Avitene. (Photo courtesy of Davol [formerly Medchem].)

gering further **platelet aggregation** into thrombi. Avitene should be applied with dry instruments only (Fig. 10–3), as it will adhere to wet surfaces. Wetting also decreases its hemostatic efficiency. In addition contact with nonbleeding surfaces should be avoided, as adhesions may result. Excess Avitene should be removed by irrigation within a few minutes. Avitene is available in powder form (in amounts of 0.5 g, 1 g, and 5 g), in sheets of various sizes, and packaged in delivery devices for endoscopic and specialty applications.

Instat MCH is derived from bovine deep flexor tendon, a source of pure collagen. The microfibrillar form allows the surgeon to grasp only the amount needed with a forceps. Onset of action is 2–4 minutes. Instat MCH is absorbable, but removal is recommended. It is available in 0.5- and 1-g containers.

OXIDIZED CELLULOSE

The hemostatic action of oxidized cellulose is not yet clearly understood. When applied to bleeding surfaces, oxidized cellulose swells, becoming a gelatinous mass which serves as a nucleus for clotting. Oxidized cellulose is absorbable, but removal is recommended after hemostasis is achieved. Oxidized cellulose comes in gauze or cotton form and is best applied when dry. The cotton form should be separated into strands or small pieces prior to use. The gauze form may be cut to desired shape and size. Oxidized cellulose is commonly used in neurosurgery and otorhinolaryngology. Examples of oxidized cellulose include Oxycel (gauze and cotton), Surgicel gauze, and Surgicel NuKnit (a knitted fabric), all available in multiple sizes (Table 10–4).

ABSORBABLE COLLAGEN SPONGE

Absorbable collagen sponges are made from purified bovine collagen. The sponge is cut to desired shape and applied with pressure to a bleeding site. When applied

Table 10–4 Surgicel and Surgicel NuKnit Sizes

Surgicel
½ × 2 inches
2 × 3 inches
2 × 14 inches
4 × 8 inches
Surgicel NuKnit
1 × 1 inches
1 × 3.5 inches
3 × 4 inches
6 × 9 inches

to bleeding surfaces, the sponge promotes platelet aggregation. Collagen may reduce the bonding strength of methyl methacrylate (bone cement), so it should not be applied to bone prior to placement of a prosthesis requiring cement fixation. Examples of absorbable collagen sponges are Collastat, Helistat, Hemopad, and Instat. One brand of collagen sponge, Superstat, contains calcium chloride. When applied, the sponge activates the body's coagulation mechanism to achieve hemostasis in 2–3 minutes. Superstat should be applied dry, then covered with a laparotomy or gauze sponge. It is contraindicated in neurosurgical applications. Superstat is available in two sizes, with calcium chloride concentrations of 1.5 and 3%.

THROMBIN

Thrombin is a topical hemostatic agent of bovine origin. It may come prepared in a spray bottle kit or in a powder form that must be reconstituted with sterile water or saline. Thrombin should be used immediately after preparation, or it should be refrigerated and used immediately after reconstituting. Thrombin works by catalyzing the conversion of fibrinogen to fibrin, thus increasing the speed of the natural clotting mechanism. Thrombin may be applied topically in solution or as a powder; however, it must never be introduced into large blood vessels, as intravascular clotting and death may result. Thrombin is measured in units rather than milligrams and comes in strengths from 1,000 to 20,000 units for different applications. The speed of thrombin's clotting action depends on the concentration used—typically 100 units per milliliter (1,000 units of thrombin with 10 mL of diluent). Concentrations as high as 2,000 units per milliliter may be used if needed. Areas of profuse bleeding, as in liver trauma, may require the highest concentration of thrombin.

BONE WAX

Bone wax is a topical hemostatic agent made from beeswax. It comes packaged for sterile delivery in a foil-type wrapper inside a peelable package. Bone wax is used primarily in orthopedics and neurosurgery to control bleeding on bone surfaces. It acts as a mechanical barrier rather than as a matrix for clotting. Bone wax is a pliable, opaque, waxy substance that is sparingly applied directly onto bone. It may harden when kept outside of the foil package for extended periods of time.

CHEMICAL HEMOSTATICS

Some hemostatic agents, such as tannic acid and silver nitrate, chemically cauterize bleeding surfaces. Tannic acid is a powder made from an astringent plant. Applied topically to mucous membranes, it helps stop capillary bleeding. Tannic acid may be used after tonsillectomy in combination with 1%

Neosynephrine (a vasoconstrictor). A tonsil sponge is saturated with the tannic acid/Neosynephrine mixture and applied to the tonsillar fossa to control minor bleeding.

Silver nitrate is another cauterizing agent, especially when mixed with potassium nitrate. This combination is molded onto applicator sticks (which come in 6- and 12-inch lengths) and used to cauterize wounds. It can also remove granulation tissue or warts. Silver nitrate sticks also come in 18-inch lengths for use with a sigmoidoscope. The applicator tips are moistened with water and applied to the desired area for treatment. Silver nitrate has a caustic effect on mucous membranes and should NOT be used around eyes. It may also discolor the treatment site with repeated application.

Systemic Coagulants

Systemic coagulants are agents that replace deficiencies in the natural clotting mechanism. If needed, systemic coagulants are usually administered preoperatively. Occasionally, a systemic coagulant may be administered intraoperatively by the anesthesia provider. Systemic coagulants may be used to replace calcium, vitamin K, or some of the coagulation factors in the blood. Such deficiencies in coagulation substances may be due to heredity, as in hemophilia, or they may be acquired, as a vitamin K deficiency. Systemic coagulants may be administered intravenously, intramuscularly, orally, or subcutaneously, depending on the medication used. See Table 10–5 for a summary of systemic coagulants.

Table 10–5 Systemic Coagulants

Calcium salts
Calcium chloride
Vitamin K
Konakion
Mephyton
AquaMephyton
Blood coagulation factors
Antihemophilic factor (VIII)
Hemofil-M
Koate-HT
Monociate
Factor IX complex
KonyneHT
Profiline Heat-treated
Proplex

CALCIUM SALTS

Calcium, which is the body's most common mineral, is critical for numerous body functions, including blood coagulation. If calcium levels fall during surgery, natural coagulation becomes less efficient, so calcium salts may be administered intravenously to assist the mechanism. During transfusions, for example, anesthesia providers must monitor blood calcium levels very closely, because the processing of donated blood tends to strip it of calcium. Typically, an injection of a 10% solution of calcium chloride ($CaCl_2$) is used to restore calcium levels intraoperatively. Calcium may also be given preoperatively. In the medical setting, calcium may be given by mouth (in tablet form) or injected intramuscularly.

☞ Calcium salts are NOT given to patients with a history of malignant hyperthermia (MH). Why? Because one aspect of MH is increased calcium release from muscle cells. (See Chapter 15.)

VITAMIN K

Vitamin K is a fat-soluble vitamin; it promotes blood clotting by increasing synthesis of prothrombin in the liver. In the surgical patient, a deficiency in vitamin K can lead to excessive bleeding. Decreased vitamin K levels are seen in patients on oral anticoagulants, such as coumarin derivatives. Some antibacterial therapies also cause vitamin K deficiency. If needed, vitamin K is administered PO, IM, or SC 24–36 hours preoperatively, because it takes several hours to produce an acceptable effect. Vitamin K is also used in the medical setting to counteract anticoagulant-induced prothrombin deficiency. It does not directly counteract oral anticoagulants, but stimulates prothrombin formation by the liver. Vitamin K will not counteract the action of heparin. Administration of vitamin K intravenously has resulted in severe anaphylactic reactions; therefore, it is given IV only when other routes are not feasible and when the risks have been recognized and considered. Vitamin K is available as phytonadione (Konakion, Mephyton, or AquaMephyton).

BLOOD COAGULATION FACTORS

Deficiency of any clotting factor interferes with effective coagulation. Two blood factors administered intravenously in the medical setting are antihemophilic factor (AHF), known as factor VIII, and factor IX complex. Factor VIII, a plasma protein essential for conversion of prothrombin to thrombin, is prepared from human blood plasma. This factor is absent in patients with hemophilia A and must be administered intravenously as needed prior to an operative procedure. Antihemophilic factor is available as Hemofil-M, Koate-HS, and Monociate. Factor IX complex is a concentrate of dried plasma fractions—mainly coagulation factors II, VII, IX, and X. Factor IX complex may be administered preoperatively as needed in patients with hemophilia B. It is also used in the medical setting to reverse coumarin-induced hemorrhage. Factor IX complex is available as Konyne-HT, Profiline Heat-treated, and Proplex.

Anticoagulants

Anticoagulants are drugs that prevent or interfere with blood coagulation. Anticoagulants are administered in the medical setting to prevent venous thrombosis, pulmonary embolism, acute coronary occlusions after myocardial infarction (MI), and strokes caused by an embolus or cerebral blood clot. Anticoagulants do not dissolve existing clots; rather, they prevent new clots from forming. A surgical patient with a history of arterial stasis, or one who must be immobilized for a prolonged period of time after surgery, may be placed on prophylactic anticoagulant therapy. Anticoagulants are used in surgery to prevent clot formation as a response to trauma or manipulation of blood vessels. Patients receiving anticoagulants are carefully monitored for signs of hemorrhage, a common side effect. Minor hemorrhage may be evident as bruising, nosebleed (epistaxis), blood in urine (hematuria), or bloody stools (melena).

Parenteral Anticoagulants

Parenteral anticoagulants (Table 10–6) are drugs administered intravenously, subcutaneously, or topically that interfere with blood clotting. Heparin sodium is the most commonly used parenteral anticoagulant. It is derived from porcine intestinal mucosa and is available in solution for injection. Heparin is measured in units rather than milligrams and is available in doses of 1,000 to 20,000 units per milliliter. Heparin works at several points in the clotting cascade by inhibiting factor X, interfering with the conversion of prothrombin to thrombin, and by inactivating thrombin, thus preventing conversion of fibrinogen to fibrin. Heparin also interferes with platelet aggregation. Onset of action is rapid, usually within 5 minutes, with duration of 2–4 hours. Adverse reactions include increased risk of hemorrhage and thrombocytopenia (decrease in platelets), so

Table 10–6 Parenteral Anticoagulants and Antidote

Anticoagulant	Antidote
Heparin sodium	Protamine sulfate
Enoxaprin sodium	Protamine sulfate

heparin is contraindicated in patients with existing severe thrombocytopenia. Coagulation studies such as PTT (see Insight 10–1) are used to monitor heparin's therapeutic action.

If a high risk of pulmonary embolism exists, heparin may be administered preoperatively by subcutaneous injection at least 1 hour prior to a surgical procedure. Heparin is the primary anticoagulant used intraoperatively. It is administered intravenously 3 minutes prior to placement of an arterial occluding clamp. Three minutes is usually sufficient to allow systemic distribution of heparin, preventing the formation of blood clots due to arterial stasis. Some types of vascular graft materials must be preclotted prior to insertion to minimize blood loss. Preclotting a graft requires saturation with blood, which must be withdrawn prior to systemic heparinization to be effective.

Heparin is frequently used from the sterile back table during peripheral vascular procedures. A dilute solution, such as 5,000 units of heparin in 1000 mL of normal saline, is used as a topical arterial irrigant. Careful attention must be paid to identifying the correct dosage, because 1 mL of heparin can contain 1,000 units, 5,000 units, 10,000 units, or 20,000 units (Table 10–7). It is the strength, not the volume, of heparin that determines the dose. The circulator and scrub must always read aloud the number of units of heparin placed in solution for irrigation, and the scrub must repeat that solution strength to the surgeon prior to passing the drug. Heparin may be used intraoperatively in many types of vascular procedures. During a femoral embolectomy, for example, heparin is administered through an irrigating arterial catheter to clear the artery of remaining clot or embolic debris. In cardiovascular procedures requiring extracorporeal circulation, heparin is administered to prevent coagulation of blood in the pump tubing. Heparin, in various strengths, is also used during placement of a venous access port or catheter. Proper identification—and careful labeling—of different strengths of heparin on the back table is mandatory (Fig. 10–4). For instance, a port or catheter may be flushed prior to insertion with a mild heparin solution, such as 10 units per milliliter; then when it's in position, it may be flushed with 100 units per milliliter. The scrubbed surgical technologist is responsible for passing the correct heparin solution at the correct time.

INSIGHT 10–1 | **BLOOD COAGULATION STUDIES**

Two laboratory tests are routinely used to assess blood coagulation. Prothrombin time (PT, pro-time) is an evaluation of the extrinsic and common coagulation system. PT is used to monitor anticoagulant therapy by vitamin K antagonists such as warfarin. PT screens for adequate amounts of factors I, II, VII, and X. Partial thromboplastin time (PTT) and activated partial thromboplastin time (APTT) evaluate the intrinsic and common coagulation pathways. PTT is used to monitor heparin therapy. PTT screens for deficiencies of all coagulation factors except VII and XIII. Laboratory results vary by method used, so are reported along with the reference range.

Table 10–7   Heparin Strengths

Strength	Volume
Vials	
1,000 units per mL	10 mL, 30 mL
5,000 units per mL	1 mL, 10 mL
10,000 units per mL	1 mL, 4 mL
Heparin in Tubex cartridges	
1,000 units/mL	1 mL
2,500 units/mL	1 mL
5,000 units/mL	1 mL
7,500 units/mL	1 mL
10,000 units/mL	0.5 mL, 1 mL
20,000 units/mL	1 mL
Heparin Lock Flush (Vials)	
10 units/mL	10 mL, 30 mL
100 units/mL	10 mL, 30 mL
Heparin Lock Flush (Tubex cartridge)	
10 units/mL	1 mL, 2.5 mL
100 units/mL	1 mL, 2.5 mL

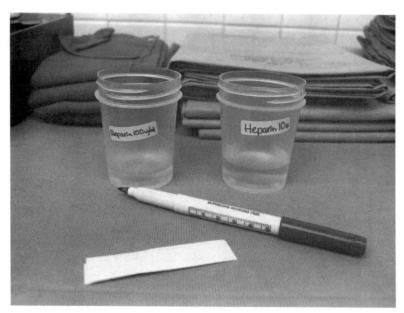

Figure 10–4   Labeled heparin solutions on sterile back table.

The antidote for heparin is protamine sulfate, a parenteral anticoagulant that inactivates heparin. Protamine may be used to treat a heparin overdose, or to reverse heparin-induced anticoagulation. Protamine is administered by slow intravenous injection. In surgery, protamine may be administered by the anesthesia provider prior to wound closure if anticoagulation is still evident.

Enoxaparin sodium (Lovenox) is a parenteral anticoagulant used to prevent postoperative deep vein thrombosis following hip or knee replacement. A sterile, low–molecular-weight heparin derived from porcine intestinal mucosa, Lovenox is administered by subcutaneous injection. A preparation of the drug can be sent home with the patient, avoiding prolonged hospitalization for anticoagulant therapy. Enoxaprin is contraindicated in patients with active major bleeding or those with hypersensitivity to heparin or pork products. It should not be given in combination with other anticoagulants, including aspirin. Side effects include local irritation, pain at the injection site, fever, and nausea. Rare adverse effects include hemorrhagic complications and thrombocytopenia. Levels of enoxaprin are monitored with a complete blood count (CBC) and platelet counts. Protamine sulfate may be administered by slow intravenous injection as an antidote to excessive enoxaparin anticoagulation.

Oral Anticoagulants

Oral anticoagulants are used for long-term management of thromboembolic disease such as deep vein thrombosis or pulmonary embolism. Oral anticoagulant therapy is also used to prevent blood clots associated with cerebrovascular thromboembolic disease. Warfarin sodium (Coumadin), a coumarin derivative, is a widely prescribed oral anticoagulant. Coumarin derivatives act by inhibiting vitamin K activity in the liver, thereby preventing formation of coagulation factors II, VII, IX, and X. Warfarin, which is highly bound to plasma proteins (see Chapter 2), is metabolized in the liver and excreted in the urine. The onset of action of warfarin is prolonged, usually 12–72 hours; and its duration is 5–7 days. The effectiveness of warfarin therapy is assessed by measuring prothrombin time (PT), which should be approximately twice normal. As drug interactions are common with warfarin, all other medications must be closely monitored. Some common side effects include hemorrhagic episodes such as epistaxis, hematuria, and bleeding gums. The antidote for excessive warfarin anticoagulation is vitamin K.

Oral anticoagulant therapy poses a particular problem when a patient requires surgical intervention. In select cases, warfarin may be temporarily discontinued approximately one week prior to an elective surgical procedure. But patients on oral anticoagulants who require emergency surgery will exhibit prolonged bleeding times. Vitamin K may be administered during surgery, but its effects may not be seen for several hours. Meticulous hemostasis is necessary to minimize blood loss in patients on oral anticoagulant therapy.

Aspirin (acetylsalicylic acid; ASA) is also considered an oral anticoagulant; it prevents clot formation by inhibiting platelet aggregation. Aspirin may be given after myocardial infarction or recurrent transient ischemic attacks (TIA) to reduce risk of further incidence. The administration of just 300 mg of aspirin can double normal bleeding time for up to seven days. Thus, if possible, patients on aspirin therapy should discontinue use at least one week prior to elective surgery.

Thrombolytics

Thrombolytics (Table 10–8) are agents given intravenously in the medical setting to help dissolve blood clots. These drugs activate plasminogen to form plasmin, which digests fibrin. And when fibrin breaks down, the clot dissolves. Thrombolytics are used to treat acute myocardial infarction when coronary artery thrombosis is present. Anticoagulant therapy may be used in conjunction with thrombolytic agents since clot formation is an ongoing process. The major side effect of thrombolytics is hemorrhage, so patients are closely monitored. Mild side effects include skin rash, itching, nausea, and headache. Streptokinase (Streptase), an enzyme produced by a strain of streptococci, and urokinase (Abbokinase), derived from human tissue, are examples of thrombolytic agents. Antistreplase (Eminase) is a combination of streptokinase and human plasminogen.

Alteplase (Activase) is a thrombolytic agent produced by recombinant DNA technology. It is a biosynthetic form of a naturally occurring enzyme, human tissue-type plasminogen activator (t-PA). Alteplase is used concurrently with heparin in treatment of acute myocardial infarction. In specific cases, altepase may also play a role in the treatment of strokes, pulmonary emboli, and peripheral vascular occlusions. Because it is a human enzyme, fewer allergic and hypersensitivity reactions occur with altepase than with other thrombolytic agents. Another advantage of altepase is its ability to act specifically—targeting clots rather than exerting systemic effects.

Table 10–8 **Thrombolytics**

Generic Name	Trade Name
Streptokinase	Streptase
Urokinase	Abbokinase
Antistreplase	Eminase
Altepase	Activase

Summary

Blood naturally contains both coagulants and anticoagulants, but anticoagulants are normally dominant because they keep blood in its flowing, liquid form. Occasionally, however, it becomes necessary for blood to solidify, or clot. Blood coagulation is a process that minimizes blood loss when small blood vessels are disrupted. The formation of a blood clot is the result of a three-stage cascade of events. Clot formation may be initiated via two different pathways—extrinsic or intrinsic. Thrombosis is the formation of a blood clot within an unbroken blood vessel. If natural coagulation or anticoagulation is inadequate, medical or surgical intervention may be necessary.

Drugs that affect blood coagulation fall into two main categories: coagulants and anticoagulants. Coagulants assist the body's natural clotting mechanism. Coagulants applied topically during surgery to control minor bleeding and capillary oozing are called hemostatics. Many varieties of hemostatics are available packaged for delivery to the sterile field. Systemic coagulants are administered in the medical setting to replace missing or inadequate levels of necessary components such as calcium, vitamin K, and some coagulation factors.

Anticoagulants work to prevent undesired clotting, slow the normal clotting mechanism, or help break up existing clots. Anticoagulants fall into three basic categories: parenteral anticoagulants, oral anticoagulants, and thrombolytics. Heparin is the most common parenteral anticoagulant used in surgery, usually during peripheral and cardiovascular procedures. Parenteral and oral anticoagulants are administered in the medical setting to prevent deep vein thrombosis, pulmonary embolism and strokes, and to treat myocardial infarction. Thrombolytics are administered intravenously to break up existing blood clots. When drugs that affect blood coagulation are administered, the patient must be carefully monitored for adverse effects.

REVIEW

1. Which hemostatic agents are used most frequently in your clinical facility? In which procedures?

2. Why are hemostatics used?

3. What are systemic coagulants used for? Can you name some?

4. Name three surgical procedures that usually require heparin ready on the back table. In which strengths?

5. How does oral anticoagulant therapy affect the patient about to undergo a surgical procedure?

6. Why are thrombolytics administered?

CHAPTER **11**

Ophthalmic Agents

Anatomy Review
Categories of Ophthalmic Agents
Enzymes
Irrigating Solutions
Viscoelastic Agents
Miotics

Mydriatics and Cycloplegics
Ointments and Lubricants
Anesthetics
Antiglaucoma Agents
Anti-inflammatory Agents
Dyes

OBJECTIVES

Upon completion of this chapter you should be able to:

1 Define terminology related to ophthalmic drugs.
2 State the purpose of each category of drugs.
3 Describe use of ophthalmic drugs in surgery.
4 List examples of drugs in each category.

KEY TERMS

Constrict To decrease in size, as in narrowing of the pupil.
Dilate To increase in size, as in enlargement of the pupil.

Glaucoma Group of ocular diseases characterized by increased intraocular pressure.

Proteolytic Pertaining to the breakdown of protein.

Ophthalmic surgical procedures often require the use of several medications from the sterile back table. Initially, the scrubbed surgical technologist must properly identify and label all medications received into the sterile field. In addition, the surgical technologist must understand the purpose of each drug in order to pass it to the surgeon at the appropriate time. In this chapter we'll focus on definitions, purposes, routes, and agents in each ophthalmic drug category used in surgery. A review of basic anatomy is included for reference.

Anatomy Review

The eye (Fig. 11–1) is a complex sense organ that receives visual stimuli and transmits signals via the optic nerve (cranial nerve II) to the brain for interpretation. Accessory structures include eyebrows, eyelids, eyelashes, and the lacrimal (tear-producing) system. A thin mucous membrane called the conjunctiva lines the inside of the eyelids and the anterior surface of the eyeball (globe). Only about

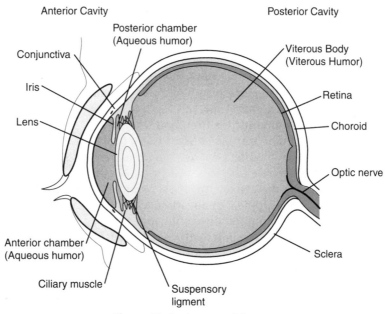

Figure 11–1 Anatomy of the eye.

17% of the globe is visible; the remainder is protected within the bony orbit. The globe consists of three layers of tissue; fibrous, vascular, and nervous. The fibrous outer coat of the eye is composed of dense, white connective tissue, called sclera. Sclera gives the globe its shape and provides protection. The cornea is made of clear, nonvascular fibrous tissue and serves as the "window" of the eye. The area where the cornea and sclera meet is called the limbus. Deep to the limbus is a venous sinus called the canal of Schlemm. The vascular layer of the eye is called choroid. The anterior, and thickest, portion of choroid is the ciliary body. The ciliary body secretes aqueous humor from structures called ciliary processes. Ciliary muscle arises in the ciliary body and attaches to the lens, altering its shape to accommodate near or distant vision. The iris is attached to the ciliary process and is positioned between the cornea and lens. The iris consists of radial and circular muscle fibers whose function is to change the size of the pupil. The pupil is an opening in the center of the iris. The pupil regulates the amount of light entering the eye by **constricting** or **dilating**. The nervous layer of the eye, called the retina, is present only posteriorly and covers the choroid. Images focused onto the retina trigger sensory receptors characterized as rods and cones. Signals are then transmitted via the optic nerve to the brain for recognition.

The lens is positioned just behind the iris and serves to focus images onto the retina. The lens consists of protein fibers arranged in onion-like layers. The lens, which is normally transparent, is covered by a clear fibrous capsule and held in place by suspensory ligaments called zonula.

The interior portion of the globe contains two cavities, anterior and posterior, separated by the lens. The anterior cavity is further separated into anterior and posterior chambers. The anterior chamber is posterior to the cornea and anterior to the iris. The posterior chamber is behind the iris and anterior to the lens. The entire anterior cavity is filled with aqueous humor (fluid) secreted by the ciliary processes. Aqueous humor flows forward in the anterior cavity and drains through the trabecular meshwork into the canal of Schlemm. If a blockage occurs in the trabecular meshwork, intraocular pressure builds, causing **glaucoma.** The posterior cavity, which is between the lens and retina, is filled with a thick substance called vitreous humor. Vitreous humor gives the globe its shape, keeps the retina in position, and contributes to intraocular pressure. Unlike aqueous humor, vitreous humor is not replaced.

The eye contains a barrier similar to the blood–brain barrier. The blood–eye barrier prevents effective absorption of most systemically administered medications. For this reason, the most common administration route for ophthalmic medications is topical application, although a few agents may be given orally or parenterally. Ophthalmic agents administered topically enter systemic circulation through the conjunctival vessels and the nasolacrimal system. About 80% of eyedrops enter the nasolacrimal system, then drain from nose to mouth and enter the stomach where absorption takes place.

Figure 11–2 illustrates proper administration of topical ophthalmic solutions. After drug administration compression of the lacrimal sac prevents rapid drainage of medication into the lacrimal system.

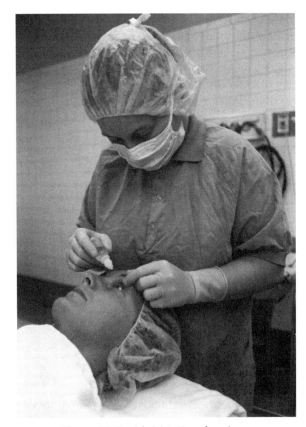

Figure 11–2 Administration of eyedrops.

Categories of Ophthalmic Agents

Enzymes

Enzymes are proteins that act as catalysts; that is, they speed up chemical reactions. Two enzymes are used in ophthalmic surgery (Table 11–1). Hyaluronidase (Wydase) is an enzyme extracted from highly purified bovine testicular hyaluronidase. Mixed with injectable local anesthetic agents, Wydase increases the rate and extent of anesthetic diffusion through tissue for nerve block. Alpha-

Table 11–1 Enzymes Used in Ophthalmology

Hyaluronidase (Wydase)	Increase diffusion of an anesthetic through tissue
Alpha-chymotrypsin (Alpha-Chymar, Zolyse)	Dissolve zonula for intracapsular cataract extraction

chymotrypsin (Alpha-Chymar, Zolyse) may be injected during intracapsular cataract extraction to break down the suspensory ligaments (zonula) holding the lens in place. Alpha-chymotrypsin is a **proteolytic** enzyme; specifically, it dissolves the protein structure of fibrous connective tissue in zonula. Newer techniques of cataract extraction—phacoemulsification and extracapsular cataract extraction—leave zonula intact, so the use of proteolytic enzymes has become less frequent.

Irrigating Solutions

Irrigating solutions are used during ophthalmic procedures to cleanse the operative site and keep the cornea moist. The most common ophthalmic irrigating solution is balanced salt solution (BSS). BSS is a sterile, physiologically balanced irrigant. It is packaged in sterile containers of 15 and 30 mL for topical use from the sterile field; it also comes in bottles of 250 and 500 mL for infusion using administration tubing sets. During most ophthalmic procedures, the scrubbed surgical technologist will periodically irrigate the cornea with BSS. Other ophthalmic irrigating solutions (A-K Rinse, Blinx, Irigate) are available for over-the-counter purchase.

Viscoelastic Agents

Viscoelastic agents are thick, jelly-like substances injected into the eye during certain ophthalmic procedures. These agents are often injected into the anterior chamber during cataract extraction to keep the chamber expanded and prevent injury to surrounding tissue. Viscoelastic agents may also be used as a vitreous substitute or tamponade (compression). Examples of viscoelastic agents (Table 11–2) include sodium hyaluronate (Healon, Amvisc-Plus), 2% hydroxypropyl methylcellulose (Occucoat), and chondroitin sulfate–sodium hyaluronate (Viscoat).

Miotics

Miotics (Table 11–3) are drugs that constrict the pupil by stimulating the sphincter muscle of the iris. Because constriction of the pupil (miosis) reduces intra-

Table 11–2 Viscoelastic Agents

Sodium hyaluronate (Healon, Amvisc-Plus)
Hydroxypropyl methylcellulose (2%) (Occucoat)
Chondroitin sulfate–sodium hyaluronate (Viscoat)

Table 11–3 Miotic Agents

Acetylcholine chloride	Miochol
Carbachol	Miostat
Pilocarpine hydrochloride	Pilocar

ocular pressure, miotics are frequently used in short-term treatment of glaucoma. Miotics may be used intraoperatively when pupillary constriction is indicated, as in laser iridectomy. Occasionally, miotics are used to maintain the position of an implanted lens after cataract extraction. Miotics may be administered by injection or topical application. Side effects include blurred vision, eye, eyebrow, or eyelid pain, abdominal cramps, and diarrhea.

Acetylcholine chloride is a miotic agent available in a solution of mannitol marketed as Miochol. It may be used for initial treatment of chronic open-angle glaucoma and acute glaucoma; this is because miosis facilitates drainage of aqueous humor. Miochol may be injected during surgery to decrease intraocular pressure, and to cause miosis if needed. Miosis will last about 10 minutes. Miochol should be reconstituted immediately before use. Carbachol (IsoptoCarbachol) is used topically to reduce intraocular pressure in glaucoma, and by injection (Miostat) into the anterior chamber as needed intraoperatively. Pilocarpine hydrochloride (Pilocar, IsoptoCarpine), in 1% and 4% ophthalmic solution, is another topical miotic. Pilocarpine (as does acetylcholine) acts directly on the smooth muscle of the iris to stimulate miosis. Pilocarpine increases flow of aqueous humor through the trabecular meshwork; thus, it is most useful in treatment of open-angle glaucoma.

Mydriatics and Cycloplegics

Both mydriatics and cycloplegics (Table 11–4) are paralytic agents used to dilate the pupil prior to ophthalmoscopy. Both kinds of agents cause *mydriasis*—dilation of the pupil—by paralyzing the sphincter muscle of the iris. Cycloplegics also paralyze the accommodation mechanism. (This means that patients may be

Table 11–4 Mydriatics and Cycloplegics

Mydriatics	
Atropine sulfate	Atropisol
Phenylephrine	Neo-Synephrine
Cycloplegics	
Cyclopentolate	Cyclogyl
Tropicamide	Mydriacyl

unable to see near objects clearly.) After topical instillation of mydriatics or cycloplegics, the lacrimal sac should be compressed for 2–3 minutes to avoid rapid systemic absorption of the medication (Fig. 11–3). Common mydriatic agents are atropine and phenylephrine. Atropine sulfate (Atropisol), a belladonna alkaloid, is available for ophthalmic use in solutions of .25% and 2%, and in ointment of .5% and 1% for topical application. Atropine may be used to dilate the pupil for a few weeks after surgery if needed. Atropine's onset is less than 15 minutes, while peak effect is seen in 30–40 minutes; duration is 7–10 days. Atropine causes some cycloplegia. Phenylephrine (Neo-Synephrine) is available in solutions of 2.5% and 10% for topical ophthalmic use. Its onset is approximately 30 minutes, with effects lasting 2–3 hours. Cycloplegic agents include cyclopentolate (Cyclogyl) and tropicamide (Mydriacyl), both available in .5% and 1% solutions.

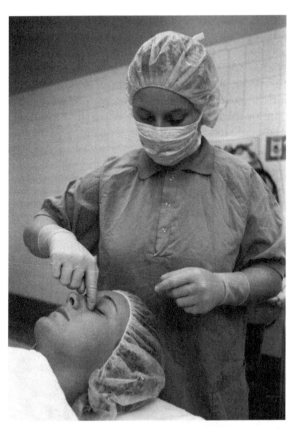

Figure 11-3 Application of pressure on lacrimal sac after administration of topical solution.

Ointments and Lubricants

Several diverse ophthalmic medications are available in ointment form. Antibiotics are frequently used in ophthalmology to treat external ocular infections and as prophylaxis against postoperative infections. Ophthalmic antibiotic preparations include aminoglycosides such as gentamycin, neomycin, and tobramycin. Interestingly, no nephrotoxicity or ototoxicity has been noted with ophthalmic use of aminoglycosides. Gentamycin (Garamycin, Genoptic) is available in .3% solution or ointment, tobramycin (Tobrex) in .3% solution or ointment, and neomycin in a solution of 2.5 mg/mL or ointment 5 mg/g. Neomycin is also available as Neosporin, combined with polymixin and bacitracin. Other common ophthalmic antibiotics include bacitracin ointment (A-K Tracin) in 500 u/g and 1000 u/g, erythromycin (Ilotycin) .5% ointment, and sulfacetamide (Sulamyd) in 10% and 30% solution and 10% ointment.

Lubricants are also available in ointment form. Ophthalmic lubricants are frequently used when a general anesthetic is administered for any surgical procedure. Under general anesthesia, eyelids are relaxed and the corneal reflex is absent. To prevent corneal drying or damage, a lubricant such as Lacrilube or Duratears is applied to each eye and the eyelids are taped closed. Upon emergence from anesthesia, patients may exhibit blurred vision; although this blurring is due to the ointment, they should be prevented from rubbing their eyes.

Combinations of antibiotics and steroids (anti-inflammatory agents) are also available in ointment form. Maxitrol ointment is neomycin and polymixin B with dexamethasone. Tobradex is tobramycin with dexamethasone.

Anesthetics

Anesthetics are drugs that interfere with normal transmission of pain impulses to the brain. Many ophthalmic surgical procedures require the use of a topical or an injected anesthetic agent (Table 11–5). Cocaine solution (1% and 4%) was the initial topical anesthetic agent used in ophthalmology; but it is used only

Table 11–5 **Ophthalmic Anesthetic Agents**

Topical
Cocaine solution (4%)
Tetracaine (Pontocaine)
Proparacaine (Alcaine, Ophthaine)

Injectable
Lidocaine (Xylocaine)
Bupivicaine (Marcaine, Sensorcaine)

rarely now. Two common topical ophthalmic anesthetics are tetracaine and proparacaine. Tetracaine (Pontocaine) is available in a 5% ophthalmic solution. Tetracaine's onset is under 1 minute, and its duration is 15–20 minutes. Proparacaine (Alcaine, Ophthaine) is available in 5% ophthalmic solution, its onset is 20 seconds, and its duration is 10–15 minutes.

Ophthalmic procedures requiring an extensive area of anesthesia are performed under a regional, retrobulbar block (see Chapter 13). Retrobulbar anesthesia, which provides both sensory and motor (movement) block, is done with a local anesthetic, such as lidocaine or bupivicaine, which is injected near the optic nerve (Fig. 11–4). Other agents may be added to the anesthetic, including hyaluronidase (Wydase) or epinephrine. Epinephrine is a powerful vasoconstrictor; it is used to prevent rapid absorption of the anesthetic, thereby prolonging the block.

Antiglaucoma Agents

Glaucoma is a general term that refers to a group of diseases characterized by increased intraocular pressure. This pressure damages the optic nerve and may cause blindness. Glaucoma results when the aqueous humor drainage mechanism is blocked. The most common form of glaucoma is chronic open-angle glaucoma. In open-angle glaucoma, the trabecular meshwork cannot drain aqueous fluid effectively. Narrow-angle glaucoma (also called angle-closure glaucoma) may be acute or chronic. This type is far rarer, comprising only about 5% of all glaucomas. Angle-closure glaucoma is caused by an abnormally narrow junction

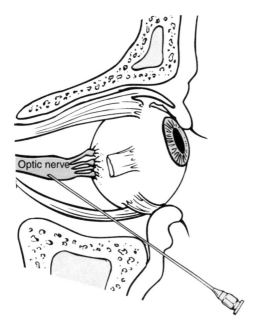

Figure 11–4   Retrobulbar block.

between the cornea and iris, blocking the flow of aqueous humor into the trabecular meshwork.

Because pupillary constriction may open the trabecular meshwork and facilitate drainage of excess fluid, short-term treatment often involves miotics. However, long-term management of increased intraocular pressure may be accomplished with several different types of agents (Table 11–6), including diuretics (see Chapter 7)—particularly carbonic anhydrase inhibitors. Carbonic anhydrase is an enzyme present in the ciliary body; it catalyzes secretion of aqueous humor. A carbonic anhydrase inhibitor like acetazolamide (Diamox) interferes with production of carbonic anhydrase; thus it reduces production of aqueous humor and decreases intraocular pressure. Acetazolamide, which reduces aqueous humor production by 50–60%, is administered orally to manage chronic open-angle glaucoma, or given intravenously to treat acute angle-closure glaucoma. With oral administration, ocular effects are seen in 1–2 hours, with a duration of 3–5 hours. Other carbonic anhydrase inhibitors include dichlophenamide (Daranide), dorzolamide (Trusopt), and methazolamide (Glauctabs).

Osmotic diuretics may also be used for short-term treatment of glaucoma. By raising the osmotic pressure of blood, osmotic diuretics cause fluid to be drawn out of the eye, lowering intraocular pressure. Ocular effects of osmotic diuretics last about 4 hours. Osmotic diuretics may be used immediately before surgery to reduce intraocular pressure, or they may be given during procedures to treat retinal detachment to aid in scleral closure. Osmotic diuretics are also

Table 11–6 Categories of Antiglaucoma Agents

Miotics

Acetylcholine chloride (Miochol)
Carbachol (IsoptoCarbachol)
Pilocarpine (Pilocar, IsoptoCarpine)

Diuretics

Carbonic anhydrase inhibitors
    Acetazolamide (Diamox)
    Dichlophenamide (Daranide)
    Dorzolamide (Trusopt)
    Methazolamide (Glauctabs)
Osmotic diuretics
    Mannitol (Osmitrol)
    Glycerine (Glyrol, Osmoglyn)
    Isorbide (Ismotic)

Beta-adrenergic blockers

Timolol (Timoptic)
Betaxolol (Betoptic)
Carteolol (Occupress)
Levobunolol (Betagan)

used in cases of acute angle-closure glaucoma to facilitate the response of the iris muscle to miotics. The most common osmotic diuretic used in ophthalmic surgery is mannitol (Osmitrol). Mannitol in a 5% to 20% solution is given intravenously in a dose of 1–2 g/kg of patient weight. For example, 500 mL of a 20% mannitol solution may be administered over a period of 3–60 minutes. When mannitol is administered preoperatively, an indwelling urinary catheter is usually inserted into the patient's bladder to accommodate resulting diuresis. Maximum effect is noted approximately an hour after administration. Other osmotic diuretics used in ophthalmology include glycerine (Glyrol, Osmoglyn) 50% solution and isorbide (Ismotic) 45% solution, both administered orally.

A group of drugs known as beta-adrenergic blockers are also used to treat glaucoma. By blocking beta-adrenergic receptor sites, these drugs reduce aqueous fluid production. Systemic side effects of beta-adrenergic blockers include decreased heart rate and blood pressure. Timolol (Timoptic) is used to treat chronic open-angle glaucoma. Although its exact mechanism not yet known, it has been reported to decrease production of aqueous humor and increase outflow. Timolol, in .25% or .5% ophthalmic solution, is administered in a dosage of one drop in the affected eye twice a day. One dose of timolol may reduce intraocular pressure for up to 24 hours. Unlike miotics, no accommodation problems are noted with use. Other beta-adrenergic blockers include betaxolol (Betoptic) .5% solution, carteolol (Occupress) 1% solution, and levobunolol (Betagan) .25% and .5% solution.

Anti-inflammatory Agents

Two categories of anti-inflammatory agents are used in ophthalmology: steroids and nonsteroidal anti-inflammatory drugs (NSAIDs). Steroids are hormones (see Chapter 9) with a wide range of effects; they are used in ophthalmology to suppress the inflammatory response to trauma. Steroids may be administered via four routes: topical, systemic, periocular, or intravitreal. Common steroids used are betamethasone (Celestone suspension), dexamethasone (Maxidex suspension, Decadron ointment and solution), and prednisolone (PredMild, PredForte suspensions).

Nonsteroidal anti-inflammatory drugs (NSAIDs) are used to reduce postoperative inflammation. Ophthalmic solutions of ketorolac .5% (Acular) and diclofenac .1% (Voltaren) are available. Nonsteroidal anti-inflammatory drugs may also be used to inhibit intraoperative miosis, particularly flurbiprofen .03% (Ocufen) and suprofen .1% (Profenal).

Dyes

Dyes are used in surgery to color or mark tissue. Ophthalmic dyes are instilled topically to diagnose abnormalities of the cornea and conjunctival epithelium or to locate foreign bodies. Dyes may also be used to observe the flow of aqueous

Table 11–7 Dyes Used in Ophthalmology

Fluorescein sodium
Rose bengal

humor or to demonstrate lacrimal system function. Examples of dyes used in ophthalmology are fluorescein sodium and rose bengal (Table 11–7). These dyes are available as individually wrapped sterile paper strips, which are moistened and applied to the anterior surface of the eye. Fluorescein sodium (Fluor-I-Strip, Ful-Glo), which is used to diagnose corneal abrasions, stains damaged or diseased corneal tissue bright green. Fluorescein sodium should not be used with soft contact lenses, because they may absorb the dye. Rose bengal in a 1% solution stains devitalized cells better than fluorescein sodium. Rose bengal is primarily used for demarcation of devitalized conjunctival epithelium seen in "dry eye" syndrome (keratoconjunctivitis sicca).

Summary

Many different drugs may be administered during ophthalmic procedures. Whether in the scrub or circulating role, the surgical technologist must be able to identify agents used routinely and recognize the purpose of each agent. The drug category usually provides information regarding the general purpose of the drug. Categories of ophthalmic drugs include enzymes, irrigating solutions, viscoelastic agents, miotics, mydriatics and cycloplegics, ointments and lubricants, anesthetics, antiglaucoma agents, anti-inflammatories, and dyes.

REVIEW

1. Why are enzymes used in ophthalmology?

2. In which ophthalmic procedures have you used an irrigating solution?

3. Which viscoelastic agent is used in your clinical facility?

4. What is the difference between a miotic and a mydriatic?

5. What types of ophthalmic medications are available in ointment form?

6. Which routes are used to administer ophthalmic anesthetics?

7. How do various antiglaucoma medications work?

8. Can you list two ophthalmic anti-inflammatory agents?

9. Why are dyes used in ophthalmology?

UNIT **THREE**

Anesthesia

Anesthesia is a complex and specialized area of pharmacology. As a surgical technologist, you'll observe the administration of anesthesia in the operating room nearly every day. Why is it necessary to learn about anesthesia at all? After all, administration of anesthetic agents is far outside the realm of the technologist's clinical practice. The fact is, understanding the terminology, methods, and agents of anesthesia will give you a more complete picture of surgical patient care. And it will make you a more effective member of the surgical team if you know the names and classification of anesthetic and supplemental agents, as well as their purposes. As team members, you'll be asked to obtain medications with whose generic and trade names you must be familiar. And to facilitate smooth flow of patient care, you'll need to understand preoperative anesthesia routines and medications. In both routine and emergency situations, all team members must contribute maximum effort in order to achieve the best possible patient outcome. For the surgical technologist, part of that effort includes learning the rudiments of pharmacology as it relates to anesthesia.

Preoperative Medications

OBJECTIVES

Upon completion of this chapter you should be able to:

1 Define terminology related to preoperative medications.
2 Identify the purposes of preoperative evaluation.
3 List classifications of preoperative medications.
4 Identify the purpose of each group of preoperative medications.
5 State examples of drugs in each classification.

KEY TERMS

Analgesic A drug or technique that reduces sensibility to pain; particularly, relief of pain without loss of consciousness.

Anesthesiologist Physician who specializes in anesthesia and the condition of patients under anesthesia.

Anesthetist A person (often a nurse) trained in administration of anesthetics.

Anticholinergic Blocking the passage of impulses from the parasympathetic nervous system; a vagolytic, parasympatholytic agent.

Aspiration Inspiration of foreign material into the airway.

CRNA Certified Registered Nurse Anesthetist

Mcg/kg Ratio representation of the amount of medication administered in micrograms per kilogram of patient body weight.

Mg/kg Ratio representation of the amount of medication administered in milligrams per kilogram of patient body weight.

Narcotic A drug that produces stupor or changes the sensibility to pain.

Opiate Any sedative narcotic containing opium or any of its derivatives.

Pulse oximeter Instrument used to measure oxygen saturation.

Preoperative preparation is necessary to maximize the safety and comfort of every surgical patient. The surgical technologist may work in a preoperative care unit or assist in preoperative preparation of patients requiring elective or emergency surgery. Surgical technologists should understand the classifications, purposes, and common pharmacologic agents used to prepare the patient for surgery in order to effectively assist the anesthesia care team.

Preoperative Evaluation

A preoperative evaluation (assessment) is performed on all surgical patients. This evaluation is conducted by a member of the anesthesia team, either an **anesthesiologist** (MD) or a **Certified Registered Nurse Anesthetist** (**CRNA**). Designed to gather pertinent patient information that can affect the course of anesthesia, the preoperative evaluation is used to confirm the patient's surgical disease and to assess concurrent medical conditions. It also lists any medications the patient may be taking, as well as allergies and physical status. Special emphasis is placed on diseases of the cardiovascular and respiratory systems and diabetes. The evaluation usually consists of a questionnaire (Fig. 12–1) to be completed by the patient and an interview with the anesthesia provider, who then completes an anesthesia evaluation form (Fig. 12–2). The patient's physical status is classified according to criteria established by the American Society of Anesthesiologists.

(Text continues on page 198.)

REGIONAL MEDICAL CENTER
PREOPERATIVE PATIENT INFORMATION (SAMPLE)

Please circle all that apply

1. Heart disease
   heart attack   chest pain   murmur
   rheumatic fever   irregular heart beat

2. High blood pressure   3. Bleeding problems

4. Lung problems
   asthma   emphysema   pneumonia
   chronic bronchitis

5. Smoking   now   ever
   How much ———————   How long ———————

6. Neurological problems
   stroke   epilepsy/seizures   nerve damage
   muscle weakness   hearing problems   balance problems
   speech problems   sight - glasses/contact lenses
   glaucoma

7. Kidney problems
   kidney failure   kidney stones   kidney infections

8. Liver problems
   hepatitis   jaundice   cirrhosis

9. Alcohol use   how much/ how often ————————————————————

10. Stomach problems   ulcers   hiatal hernia

11. Teeth: loose   chipped   caps
                        dentures   partial plate

12. Diabetes   13. Thyroid problems   14. Arthritis

15. Cancer   16. Pregnant   17. Allergies

18. Medications ——

19 Previous surgeries ————————————————————————————————————

20. Problems with anesthesia   self   family

21. Any questions?

Patient signature   Date   Time

Figure 12–1 Sample preoperative questionnaire.

REGIONAL MEDICAL CENTER
PREOPERATIVE ANESTHESIA EVALUATION (SAMPLE)

Patient name
DOB/ age
Identification number

Surgeon_____
Scheduled Procedure_____
Date of Surgery_____

HT_____   WT_____   BP_____   Temp_____   HR_____   Resp_____

H&P in chart _____   Labs complete_____   EKG _____   Chest x-ray_____

System review
Circulatory_____   History negative_____
Respiratory_____   History negative_____
CNS_____   History negative_____
Renal _____   History negative_____
Hepatic_____   History negative_____
Gastrointestinal_____   History negative_____
Endocrine_____   History negative_____
Musculoskeletal _____   History negative_____

Cancer Y   N   Pregnant Y   N
Previous anesthesia problems Y   N _____
Family anesthesia problems   Y   N _____

Physical Status   1   2   3   4   5   Emergency

Risks/alternatives addressed _____
Patients agrees to: general_____   MAC_____   Regional_____

Preoperative medications ordered:

Pre-anesthesia note:

Time   Date   Evaluator
_____   _____   _____

Post-anesthesia note:

No apparent anesthesia complications _____
Time   Date   Anesthesia staff
_____   _____   _____

Figure 12–2   Sample anesthesia evaluation form.

Preoperative Medications

During the preoperative evaluation, the MD or CRNA will determine the patient's need for preoperative medications. Some preoperative medications are given to prepare the patient physically, and some to prepare the patient psychologically. Preoperative medications can be classified by action, each group having a specific purpose.

Sedatives and Tranquilizers

Sedatives and tranquilizers are given to relieve anxiety, which is common in surgical patients. In most patients, these drugs produce a mild drowsiness, and they may have amnesiac and antiemetic effects. The most common sedatives used preoperatively are the *benzodiazepines,* which induce amnesia and relieve anxiety. Diazepam (Valium), lorazepam (Ativan), and midazolam (Versed) are all benzodiazepines. *Phenothiazines* are primarily used to treat psychotic disorders; but in low doses, they may be administered preoperatively both for their sedative and their antiemetic effects.

Diazepam is usually given intravenously as a premedication in doses of .05 to .2 **mg/kg**, with onset in less than 2 minutes. Effects will peak in 3–4 minutes and should last from 30 minutes to 2 hours. The usual dose of lorazepam for preoperative sedation is .01 to .03 mg/kg IV. Onset is between 1 and 5 minutes, with peak effect in 15–20 minutes. Effects of lorazepam may last from 6 to 24 hours. Midazolam is administered in doses of .02 to .1 mg/kg IV. Effects are seen in 1–5 minutes, peak between 5 and 30 minutes, and last from 2 to 6 hours. See Table 12–1 for a comparison of benzodiazepines used preoperatively.

A phenothiazine such as promethazine (Phenergan) may be given as a preoperative medication because of its sedative and antiemetic effects. Other sedatives also have antiemetic properties. Antihistamines, such as hydroxyzine (Vistaril) and diphenhydramine (Benadryl), produce dose-related sedation; they also reduce nausea and vomiting. Droperidol (Inapsine) is primarily an antiemetic, but it also produces sedation (see antiemetics).

Table 12–1 Comparison of Benzodiazepines Used Preoperatively

Generic Name	Trade Name	Dose (mg/kg)	Onset (min)	Peak (min)	Duration (hours)
Diazepam	Valium	0.05–0.2	<2	3–4	0.5–2
Lorazepam	Ativan	0.01–0.03	1–5	15–20	6–24
Midazolam	Versed	0.02–0.1	1–5	5–30	2–6

Narcotic Analgesics

Narcotic analgesics are used preoperatively to relieve pain and reduce the amount of anesthesia needed for surgery. The narcotic analgesic group can be further subdivided into **opiates** (derived from the opium poppy) and *synthetic narcotics* (chemically synthesized). All opiates and synthetic narcotics have certain features in common; that is they are chemically similar. All narcotics cause analgesia and mild sedation in usual doses. Nausea and vomiting are frequent side effects. Slowing of respiration and reduced intestinal motility are expected. Because of slowed respiration, supplemental oxygen may be given and monitored with a **pulse oximeter.** The patient's level of consciousness should be assessed frequently.

Morphine (Astramorph, Duramorph) is an opiate that is frequently used preoperatively. Morphine is given IV in doses of 2.5–15 mg, depending on the patient's ability to tolerate the drug. Onset of action is expected in 2–5 minutes, with peak in 5–20 minutes, and effects often last well over 2–4 hours.

The most common synthetic narcotics are meperidine (Demerol) and fentanyl (Sublimaze). Meperidine is administered IV in doses of 0.5–2 mg/kg to provide preoperative analgesia. Onset occurs in under 1–3 minutes, peak at 5–20 minutes. Meperidine provides analgesia for 2–4 hours. Fentanyl is 75–125 times more potent than morphine; it's characterized by rapid onset (30 seconds) and short duration (30 – 60 minutes). It is administered in doses of 0.7–2 **mcg/kg** preoperative analgesia. See Table 12–2 for a comparison of narcotic analgesics used preoperatively.

Narcotic analgesics are covered under federal and state controlled substances acts (see Chapter 3) and must be handled according to hospital policy. The surgical technologist must be thoroughly familiar with institutional procedures regarding controlled substances.

Anticholinergic (Antimuscarinic) Drugs

Anticholinergic drugs are used for several purposes preoperatively. These medications block certain receptors on the vagus nerve, so they are used to inhibit

Table 12–2 Comparison of Narcotic Analgesics Used Preoperatively

Generic Name	Trade Name	Dose (per kg)	Onset (min)	Peak (min)	Duration (hours)
Morphine	Astramorph	2.5–15 mg	2–5	5–20	>2
Meperidine	Demerol	0.5–2 mg	1–3	5–20	2–4
Fentanyl	Sublimaze	0.7–2 mcg	0.5	5–15	0.5–1

Table 12–3 Comparison of Anticholinergics Used Preoperatively

Generic Name	Trade Name	Dose (mg/kg)	Onset (min)	Duration (hours)
Atropine	Atropine	0.4–1.0	immediate	1–2
Glycopyrrolate	Robinul	0.2–0.4	1	2–3

mucous secretions of the respiratory and digestive tract and increase heart rate. They also serve as bronchodilators. Anticholinergics may be used to reduce the vagal response (slowed heart rate) to certain stimuli such as stretching the peritoneum or pulling on eye muscles. The two anticholinergics most frequently used preoperatively are atropine and glycopyrrolate (Robinul). Atropine is given IV in doses of .4–1.0 mg; onset is almost immediate and duration is 1–2 hours. Glycopyrrolate is administered preoperatively IV in doses of .2 to .4 mg, onset occurring within 1 minute and lasting 2–3 hours. See Table 12–3 for a comparison of anticholinergic drugs used preoperatively.

Antacids

Antacids are administered preoperatively to neutralize the acidity of stomach contents (gastric acid normally has an acidity, or pH, of 2) or to block production of gastric acid. If the patient vomits during anesthesia, the acidic gastric contents may be **aspirated** (inspired) into the lungs, causing a potentially fatal condition called aspiration pneumonia. Antacids that reduce the acidity of gastric contents minimize the amount of damage that may be caused by such aspiration. Sodium citrate with citric acid (Bicitra) is the most frequently used preoperative oral antacid. Sodium citrate is metabolized to sodium bicarbonate—a base that neutralizes gastric acid. Sodium citrate is given orally in doses of 15–30 mL (Fig. 12–3). Effects are immediate and the duration is approximately 2 hours.

Antacids may also block the production of gastric acid by parietal cells (see Chapter 8); such antacids are called histamine (H2) receptor antagonists or blockers. The two most common H2 blockers given preoperatively are cimetidine (Tagamet) and ranitidine (Zantac). Cimetidine is given intravenously as a preoperative medication in a dose of 7.5 mg/kg. Effects occur within 4–5 minutes and last approximately 4 hours. Ranitidine is administered preoperatively IV, 50 mg, with effects occurring within 15 minutes and lasting 6–8 hours.

Antiemetics

Antiemetics are administered preoperatively to reduce nausea and minimize the possibility of vomiting. Droperidol (Inapsine) is an antiemetic drug with sedative

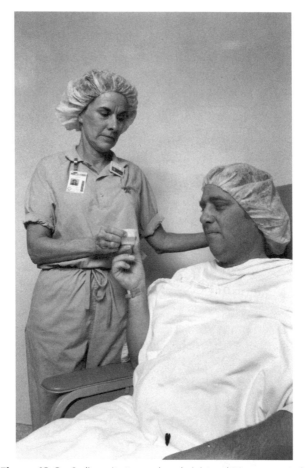

Figure 12–3 Sodium citrate may be administered PO preoperatively.

properties. It is administered intravenously, 15 mcg/kg, with effects in 3–10 minutes and duration of 2–4 hours.

Metoclopramide (Reglan) is a gastrointestinal motility agent given preoperatively for its antiemetic effects. It stimulates motility of the upper gastrointestinal tract without stimulating gastric acid secretion. Metoclopramide is administered intravenously, 10 mg, with onset expected in 1–3 minutes and duration of 1–2 hours.

Ondansetron (Zofran), an antiemetic developed for patients undergoing chemotherapy, has been found to be effective as a postoperative antiemetic as well. Ondansetron is administered IV, 4 mg, to prevent postoperative nausea and vomiting. It is effective in 5–10 minutes and lasts approximately 8 hours.

Table 12–4 **Gastric Drugs Used Preoperatively**

Generic Name	Trade Name	Dose	Onset (min)	Duration (hours)
Antacid				
Sodium citrate	Bicitra	15–30 mL	immediate	2
Cimetidine	Tagamet	7.5 mg/kg	4–5	4
Ranitidine	Zantac	50 mg	15	6–8
Antiemetic				
Droperidol	Inapsine	15 mcg/kg	3–10	2–4
Ondansetron HCl	Zofran	4 mg	5–10	8
Metoclopramide	Reglan	10 mg	1–3	1–2

Ondansetron does not stimulate gastrointestinal motility. See Table 12–4 for a summary of gastric drugs used preoperatively.

Summary

A preoperative assessment is made by the anesthesia team to determine both the appropriate anesthetic method and the preoperative medications needed. There are several general categories of medications used to prepare the patient both physically and psychologically for surgery. These include sedatives and tranquilizers, narcotic analgesics, anticholinergics, and several types of gastrointestinal drugs. The surgical technologist should be familiar with drugs administered preoperatively and their purposes in order to assist the anesthesia care team.

REVIEW

1. Why is a preoperative evaluation conducted?

2. What are the five categories of preoperative medications?

3. What is the purpose of each of the following types of drugs?
sedatives and tranquilizers   narcotic analgesics
anticholinergics   antacids
antiemetics   H2 blockers

4. State an example of a drug in each of the categories listed in question 3.

Intraoperative Anesthesia

OBJECTIVES

Upon completion of this chapter you should be able to:

1 Define terminology related to anesthesia.
2 Describe the major types of anesthesia and list applications for each type.
3 Recognize common agents used in local and regional anesthesia.
4 Compare and contrast local anesthesia and MAC.
5 Describe types of regional blocks and give an application for each type.
6 Explain the four basic components of a general anesthetic.
7 Describe methods of providing general anesthesia.

8 Define the phases of general anesthesia.

9 List agents used for induction and maintenance of general anesthesia.

10 Match generic and trade names of drugs used in anesthesia.

11 Match agents with the phase of anesthesia in which they are administered.

12 Compare and contrast depolarizing and nondepolarizing muscle relaxants.

KEY TERMS

Amnesia Impairment of memory.

Analgesia Reduction of sensibility to pain; particularly, the relief of pain without loss of consciousness.

Anesthesia Loss of feeling or sensation.

Barbiturate Any of a group of organic compounds derived from barbituric acid; used to induce sedation or sleep or to treat epilepsy.

Bradycardia Slowed heart rate.

Dura mater The outermost fibrous membrane surrounding the spinal cord.

Electrocardiogram (EKG, ECG) A tracing of the heart's electrical activity.

Endotracheal tube An airway catheter inserted in the trachea to assure patency of the upper airway and provide ventilation.

End-tidal CO_2 Measurement of expired carbon dioxide.

Exsanguinate To render bloodless.

Extubate Remove a previously inserted endotracheal tube.

Fasciculation Small local involuntary muscular contraction visible under the skin.

Flaccidity Relaxed state; absence of muscle tone.

Hypovolemic Having abnormally low volume of circulating blood in the body.

Intrathecal Within a sheath; usually, insertion through the dura of the spinal cord into the subarachnoid space.

Intubation Insertion of an endotracheal tube.

Laryngoscope An endoscope equipped with a light to enable direct examination of the larynx.

Narcosis Nonspecific reversible state of central nervous system depression marked by stupor or insensibility; induced by an opiate or narcotic.

Ophthalmologist Physician who specializes in defects, injuries, and diseases of the eye.

Plexus A network of nerves.

Rhytidectomy Plastic surgery to reduce wrinkles from the skin of the face.

Tachycardia Abnormally rapid heart rate.

Vasoconstrictor A stimulus that causes narrowing of blood vessels.

Anesthesia literally means "without sensation." The patient may be conscious or unconscious, but while receiving anesthesia, he or she will not perceive pain. The discovery of drugs that produce anesthesia (Insight 13–1) dramatically changed the practice of surgery. The precise chemicophysiologic means by which anesthetics work is not yet fully clear; but we do know that the mechanism depends on the type of drug being administered. Some drugs, for instance, induce amnesia while others induce unconsciousness or change the perception of pain. Transmission of pain sensation through nerve impulses may also be interrupted at several locations. Thus, there are various methods of accomplishing anesthesia. Three major types of anesthesia are local, regional blockade, and general.

Local Anesthesia

A local anesthetic is administered to the immediate surgical site. Whether injected into tissue or applied topically to mucosal membranes, it affects a small, circumscribed area. Local anesthetics, such as lidocaine, interfere with sensory nerve endings in the operative area; thus, they block transmission of pain impulses to the brain. When local anesthesia is used, no dedicated anesthesia provider is present to monitor the patient's vital signs during surgery. It is, however, imperative that a registered nurse (RN) be assigned to monitor the patient during the surgical procedure. The RN assesses the patient's physical condition and psychological status so that appropriate measures can be taken to maintain patient safety and comfort. Heart rate and electrical activity are measured by **electrocardiogram (ECG, EKG)**, while blood pressure, respirations, and oxygen saturation are monitored continuously. The RN may also administer sedatives as ordered by the surgeon. Only physically healthy and psychologically stable patients are appropriate candidates for local anesthesia without monitoring by anesthesia personnel.

Applications

Local anesthesia without anesthesia provider standby has several applications. In general surgery, local injections are appropriate for excision or biopsy of small soft tissue masses such as lipomas, moles, or lesions. In orthopedic surgery, local anesthesia is used for limited work on digits, such as repair of finger lacerations or toenail excisions. Local injection is used in otorhinolaryngology and plastic surgery for minor facial procedures, such as excision of lesions, and for nasal procedures such as septoplasty. In urology, cystoscopy may be performed with a topical anesthetic agent. Because local anesthesia blocks sensory nerve impulses only at the site of injection or application, the patient cannot feel pain in that area, but is still able to move muscles and feel pressure.

INSIGHT 13–1 | **YESTERDAY AND TODAY: ANESTHESIA**

In today's world, surgery and anesthesia are inseparable concepts. However, this was not always true. Surgery can actually be divided into two eras: preanesthesia and postanesthesia. In the preanesthesia era, surgery was based upon speed as the patient would often die from hemorrhage, shock, or the trauma of the operation. Ironically, shock may have helped to relieve some of the pain before death occurred. The postanesthesia era began in the 19th century when discoveries were finally published, accepted, and utilized.

Attempts to alleviate pain probably date back as far as humankind has experienced suffering. These first attempts treated pain as an evil spirit or demon and the idea was to frighten it away. Thus, early anesthesia involved tatooes, jewelry, talismans, amulets, and charms. Pain relievers existed and were used in ancient times, but they were impure, unsafe, and unreliable. Ancient pain remedies documented include a Babylonian clay tablet from approximately 2250 BC (BCE) which gives the remedy for a tooth ache. Early Egyptian surgeons applied pressure to nerves or blood vessels which caused insensibility to a specific part of the body for an operation.

Many early methods of pain control utilized drugs. Alcohol was often used in the form of spirits or wines. Along with opium and marijuana, ancient literature contains many references to the mandragora (or mandragon) plant as a pain reliever which produced a confused mental state. Dioscorides, a first-century Greek physician, administered the mandragora root boiled in wine to his patients before they went under his knife. Mandragora was also known as the "potion of the condemned" as it was given to criminals to decrease the agonies of crucifixion.

Besides drugs, there were other pain-control methods used in the preanesthesia era. One method was to produce unconsciousness by compressing the carotid arteries to decrease heart rate, or placing a wooden bowl over the patient's head and striking the bowl to cause a concussion. Another method came from China in the form of acupuncture which decreased pain sensations. A third method was cryothermia. This was documented in England in 1050 by an Anglo-Saxon manuscript which instructed the surgeon to wait awhile before making the incision as the patient sat in cold water "until it can become deadened."

The word *anesthesia* comes from the Greek word *anaisthesis* which means "no sensation." *Anesthesia* appeared in *Bailey's English Dictionary* in 1721. However, the term itself was reportedly coined by Oliver Wendell Holmes in a letter in 1846.

Unfortunately, many agents with anesthetic properties were known for generations but were not applied in surgery. The great alchemist, Paracelsus (1493?–1541), mixed sulfuric acid with alcohol and distilled his concoction. He believed this mixture, called sweet vitriol, could quiet suffering and relieve pain. We know Paracelsus's mixture today as ether. Nitrous oxide was discovered by Joseph Priestly in 1772. However, both nitrous oxide and ether were popularized by traveling "professors" as entertainment tools. Volunteers would inhale the gases and become intoxicated. This fad produced "laughing gas parties" and "ether frolics." Little known to the public at the time was the fact that a man named Humphrey Davy had described the use of nitrous oxide to relieve pain produced by a wisdom tooth in 1800.

It was after one of these public demonstrations of ether that a young physician named Crawford W. Long contemplated its use as an anesthetic during surgery. He was inspired when he saw friends receive injuries without pain while under the vapor's influence. So, on March 30, 1842, Dr. Long administered ether to James M. Venable and successfully removed a tumor from the patient's neck. A dentist named Horace Wells observed a similar demonstration of nitrous oxide in 1844 and used it in his dental practice for many years to relieve pain from tooth extractions. Unfortunately, Wells's demonstration to Harvard Medical School was not a success, possibly due to incomplete administration of the gas, and nitrous oxide was not accepted. Wells's partner, Dr. William T.G. Morton, realized that while nitrous oxide was unreliable, an alternative could be found in ether vapor. After numerous experiments, Morton contacted Dr. John Warren, a senior surgeon of the Massachusetts General Hospital. A demonstration was arranged for October 16, 1846. This demonstration was a success as a tumor was removed from the jaw of a 20–year-old male who remained insensible throughout the procedure. Thus the postanesthesia era was officially accepted with Dr. Warren's famous remark, "Gentlemen, this is no humbug."

The widespread use of anesthesia began in England on April 7, 1853, when Queen Victoria accepted the use of chloroform during childbirth. Her physician was Dr. Sir James Young Simpson. Chloroform had been discovered in 1831; however, its use by the Queen led to its acceptance by the medical community. From these beginnings, anesthesia has developed into the vital branch of medicine we know today.

Agents

Cocaine is a naturally occurring alkaloid derived from coca leaves. It has long been known to have a numbing effect when used topically on mucous membranes. Today, it is used frequently in nasal surgery. Note, however, that cocaine is for topical use only: it is never injected. Cocaine comes in 4% and 10% solutions; thus it may be administered on cotton applicators or nasal packing, or it may be sprayed directly on the mucosal surface.

In addition to its anesthetic properties, cocaine is also a powerful **vasoconstrictor.** This means it reduces bleeding and helps shrink mucous membranes. Thus it's particularly useful in nasal surgery because it allows better visualization in the nasal cavity. It also means that dosage is critical. Dosages must be carefully calculated, both to the patient's age and physical condition, using the lowest dose necessary to achieve the required anesthetic effect. The fatal overdose has been calculated at 1.2 g; however, severe toxic effects have been reported at doses as low as 20 mg. Adverse effects are seen primarily in the central nervous system. These include excitement and/or depression, and may lead to respiratory arrest.

☞ Cocaine is a controlled substance. It should never be left unattended in the operating room, and any cocaine solution dispensed but unused should be returned to the pharmacy or destroyed. At least two persons should witness the destruction of unused cocaine to verify that it has not been used for illicit purposes (see Chapter 3).

Most local anesthetics used today are not naturally occurring like cocaine. Rather, they are chemically altered or wholly synthetic compounds designed for certain desirable effects. Of these, the most common is lidocaine (Xylocaine), which is classified chemically as an amide compound. Lidocaine is fast-acting and rapidly metabolized. The duration of anesthesia with infiltrated lidocaine is 30-60 minutes. If epinephrine (see Chapter 9) is added, its effects will last from 2 to 6 hours. (Epinephrine causes vasoconstriction, thereby slowing removal of lidocaine from the injection site.) Lidocaine comes in solutions of .5%, 1%, 1.5%, and 2%, with and without epinephrine.

☞ Many people mistakenly refer to lidocaine as "Novocain," which is a completely different agent. Novocain is the trade name for procaine, which was used by dentists for many years, but is seldom used currently. Procaine is classified chemically as an ester-type anesthetic. Ester-type anesthetics cause more allergic reactions than amide-type anesthetics. Patients who are allergic to Novocain do not usually have allergies to lidocaine because these agents have different chemical structures.

Bupivicaine (Marcaine, Sensorcaine) is about four times more potent than lidocaine and has a longer duration, up to 4 hours. Bupivicaine comes in several dilutions, .25%, .5%, and .75%, with and without epinephrine 1 : 200,000.

Mepivacaine (Carbocaine, Polocaine) is about twice as potent as lidocaine, with slightly longer duration (45–90 minutes). Mepivacaine comes in 1%, 1.5%, 2%, and 3% solution and may be combined with epinephrine.

Adverse reactions to local anesthetics are primarily dose-related and affect both the central nervous system and the cardiovascular system. See Table 13–1 for a comparison of maximum dosages of local anesthetics. Adverse central nervous system effects are variable, from drowsiness at low doses to excitement or agitation at higher doses. Excitement may or may not occur, and the patient may go from a drowsy state to unconsciousness and into respiratory arrest. Nausea and vomiting may also occur. Cardiovascular adverse effects are also dose-related and include hypotension, **bradycardia** (slowed heart rate), and ventricular arrhythmias leading to possible cardiac arrest.

Table 13-1 **Maximum Dosages of Local Anesthetics for Infiltration**

Agent	Concentration	Volume (mL)	Weight (mg)
Lidocaine	.5%	up to 60	up to 300
Bupivicaine	.25%		
without epinephrine		up to 70	up to 175
with epinephrine		up to 90	up to 225
Mepivacaine	1%	up to 40	up to 400

The vasoconstricting action of epinephrine prevents an anesthetic from being carried away by the bloodstream rapidly. Thus, epinephrine may already be combined with local anesthetics, usually in concentrations of 1:50,000, 1:100,000, or 1:200,000 units. It is also available separately in the relatively high concentration of 1:1000. It is critical to administer epinephrine in the correct concentration. If the high 1:1000 concentration of epinephrine is inadvertently administered, severe **tachycardia** (rapid heart rate) and hypertension will result, increasing the potential for cardiac arrest. Using vials of local anesthetic agents with premixed epinephrine helps to prevent such errors.

See Table 13–2 for a comparison of common local anesthetic agents.

Monitored Anesthesia Care

Monitored anesthesia care (MAC) is the use of a topical or injected local anesthetic agent with the assistance of an anesthesia provider whose task it is to monitor the patient. MAC is used when the surgical procedure is more complex than those listed under local anesthesia, and often when the patient requires some sedation. Common applications for MAC include **rhytidectomy** (facial plastic surgery to reduce wrinkles), pacemaker insertion, venous access port or catheter insertion, or placement of a dialysis access graft. The anesthesia provider monitors patient's heart rate and EKG, blood pressure, respirations, and oxygen saturation continuously. In some cases, the anesthesia provider must also administer supplemental sedation or pain control to ensure that the patient is relaxed and comfortable. Common sedatives and narcotics include midazolam (Versed), fentanyl (Sublimaze), alfentanil (Alfenta), meperidine (Demerol), and propofol (Diprivan).

Regional Anesthesia

Regional anesthesia blocks nerves (not just nerve endings) at specific locations; thus, it provides a larger anesthetized area. Whereas local anesthesia involves

Table 13-2 Comparison of Common Local Anesthetic Agents

Generic Name	Trade Name	Solutions Available	Duration (hours)
Cocaine	Cocaine	4%, 10%	.5–2
Lidocaine	Xylocaine	.5%, 1%, 1.5%, 2%	.5–1
with epinephrine			2–6
Bupivicaine	Marcaine		
	Sensorcaine	.25%, .5%, .75%	4
Mepivacaine	Carbocaine		
	Polocaine	1%, 1.5%, 2%, 3%	.75–1.5

injection of a local anesthetic at the operative site, regional anesthesia involves injecting a local anesthetic into the nerves that supply the operative region. Regional blocks affect both the sensory and motor nerve supply, so an anesthetized limb becomes immobile as well as numb. Regional blocks are effective for many types of surgical procedures.

Applications

The types of regional anesthetic techniques are named for the areas of the body to be blocked. Although nearly any group of nerves can be blocked, we'll discuss only the most frequently used regional anesthetic techniques in this text.

SPINAL ANESTHESIA

In spinal anesthesia, agents are injected **intrathecally,** i.e., through the **dura mater**, into the subarachnoid space, usually in the lumbar area of the spine (Fig. 13–1). This technique anesthetizes the entire lower body. The circulator commonly assists the anesthesia provider during injection of a spinal anesthetic by helping the patient to get into optimum position (Fig. 13–2). The patient may be positioned laterally to facilitate correct needle placement. That is, patients may lie on their

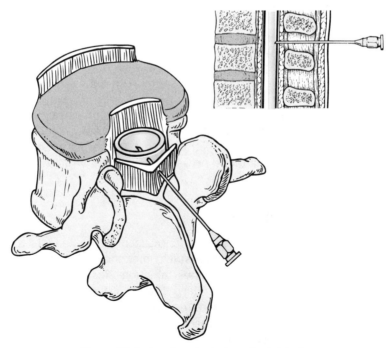

Figure 13-1 Location of spinal anesthesia injection.

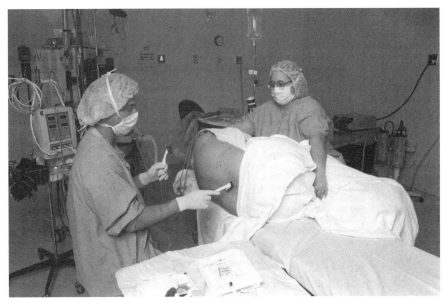

Figure 13-2   Patient positioned laterally for spinal administration.

sides, with knees bent and chin on chest. Thus, the patient is usually instructed to "curl up" as much as possible, pushing his or her lower back out toward the anesthesia provider. This position spreads the vertebral bodies apart so the spinal needle may be more easily inserted. It is, however, difficult for some patients, especially the elderly, to curl their backs. These patients may be assisted gently into position, using caution to avoid injury. Alternatively, patients may be in a sitting position for administration of a spinal anesthetic (Fig. 13–3). The patient may sit on the operating bed with his or her back to the anesthesia provider.

Spinal anesthesia is often used for transurethral resection of the prostate gland or bladder tumors, for lower leg vascular procedures such as embolectomy, and for Cesarean sections. Most local anesthetics can be used for spinal injection. A drop in blood pressure may occur with administration of a spinal or epidural anesthetic due to vasodilation.

EPIDURAL ANESTHESIA

In epidural anesthesia, an anesthetic agent is injected into the space surrounding the dura mater (Fig. 13–4). A single injection may be administered, or a catheter may be placed for continuous injection. Positioning for administration of an epidural anesthetic is identical to that described for a spinal anesthetic. Epidural anesthesia is used to relieve the pain of labor and vaginal delivery, as well as to provide anesthesia for Cesarean section. Epidural blocks may also be used as an adjunct to general anesthesia to minimize the amount of agents needed; they may also be used for postoperative pain control after such procedures as thoracotomy.

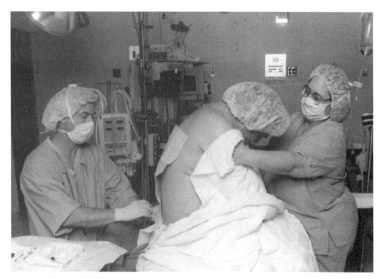

Figure 13-3 Patient in a sitting position for spinal administration.

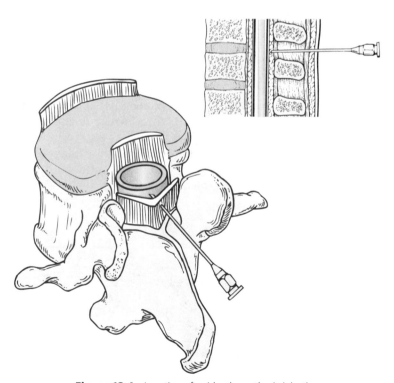

Figure 13-4 Location of epidural anesthesia injection.

CAUDAL BLOCK

Caudal anesthesia is a type of epidural block injected into the epidural space via the sacral canal (Fig. 13–5); it is primarily used to control the pain of vaginal childbirth. Caudal blocks are usually administered in the obstetrical unit rather than in the surgical suite.

RETROBULBAR BLOCK

Retrobulbar blocks are injected behind the eye into the muscle cone (Fig. 13–6). These blocks are used for many eye procedures, especially cataract extraction, because they provide a motionless, anesthetized eye. Retrobulbar blocks may be administered by an **ophthalmologist** or an anesthesia provider. A sedative may be given intravenously prior to retrobulbar injection to minimize patient discomfort.

EXTREMITY BLOCK

There are many techniques for extremity (distal arms and legs; particularly, the hand and fingers, foot and toes) block. These techniques vary, depending on the anesthesia provider's expertise and preference; but, in practice, the upper extremities (arm, hand, fingers) are more frequently blocked than the lower extremities. The arm may be blocked at several locations—including the median, radial, and ulnar nerve—while the leg may be blocked at the femoral, obturator, or tibial nerves. Depending on the surgical site, portions of the hand, foot, and digits may also be blocked.

In some cases, the arm is blocked via the axillary approach (at the armpit) at the brachial **plexus** (a network of nerves that serve the arm). In this case, the entire arm is numbed and immobilized when an anesthetic is injected into the tissue surrounding the brachial plexus, as shown in Figure 13–7. Because it's important not to penetrate the nerve sheath or damage nearby blood vessels when performing this technique, a needle attached to a nerve stimulator is inserted first. This allows the anesthesia provider to precisely locate the nerves

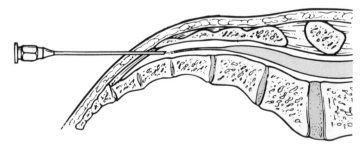

Figure 13-5   Location of caudal block.

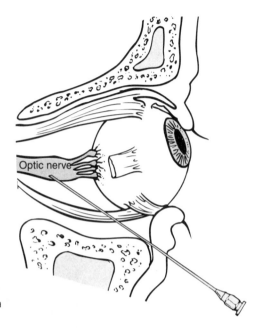

Figure 13-6 Location of retrobulbar anesthesia injection.

of the brachial plexus. This technique is used for manipulation and casting of fractures in patients who present a high risk for complications of general anesthesia; thus, it's a favored technique for use in alcohol-intoxicated patients whose central nervous system is already depressed.

Bier block, or intravenous block, is a technique that involves preliminary **exsanguination**—that is, the extremity is first rendered bloodless by constriction and elevation. This technique can be employed for procedures on upper

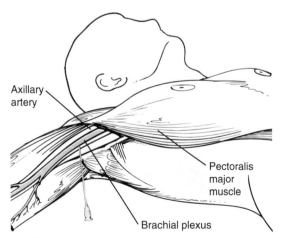

Figure 13-7 Location of axillary block injection.

and lower distal extremities, although it is most frequently used for procedures on hands (such as release of carpal tunnel, trigger finger, or Dupuytren's contracture). It is seldom used for fracture reduction, due to the discomfort occasioned by exsanguination. For a procedure on the hand, for example, a pneumatic or electric tourniquet is placed around the proximal (upper) arm. An intravenous catheter is inserted in a vein of the hand and blood is forced from the distal limb by wrapping the arm with a rubber bandage (Fig. 13–8). The tourniquet is then inflated, the bandage is removed, and a local anesthetic is injected into the catheter. The tourniquet remains inflated throughout the procedure to keep the anesthetic agent in the area. Once the surgical procedure is completed, the tourniquet is released slowly to avoid rapid infusion of the anesthetic into the systemic circulation. Bier block is both rapid and effective; but there may be some discomfort caused by exsanguination and tourniquet

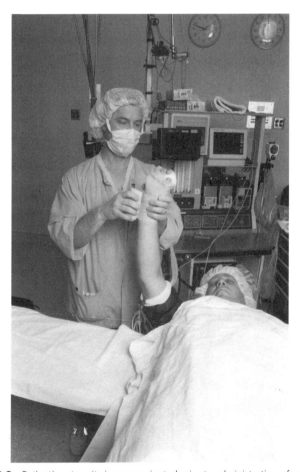

Figure 13-8   Patient's extremity is exsanguinated prior to administration of a Bier block.

use. Often, the patient requires mild sedation. In addition, use of a double cuff tourniquet provides some relief of discomfort, as the second cuff can be inflated so the first cuff can be released.

Regional extremity blocks have one primary disadvantage—it takes time for them to take effect. This means they may delay surgery. Extremity blocks may therefore be administered in the preoperative holding area. However, it is difficult to time the block so that the patient is ready when the operating room becomes available.

Any type of regional anesthesia requires continuous monitoring of the patient's vital functions, including heart rate and EKG, blood pressure, respirations, and oxygen saturation.

General Anesthesia

Many different classes of drugs have been used to achieve general anesthesia, often in combination. The desired effect is a patient who (1) remains unresponsive during surgery, (2) retains no memory of the event, and (3) maintains normal cardiovascular function. While several theories have been suggested, the exact mechanism of general anesthesia is still not clearly understood. General anesthesia is believed to interfere with the brain's ability to process pain impulses, resulting in systemic anesthesia. In the past, several drugs used to produce general anesthesia had unwanted side effects—they were extremely toxic to the patient or they were explosive. However, recent advances in anesthesia research and development have produced many new drugs that accomplish anesthesia with a high degree of safety.

Applications

The decision to use a general anesthetic is based both on the surgical procedure to be performed and on the individual patient. For instance, a general anesthetic is used when there are multiple operative sites, or for a procedure on an area that is difficult to block regionally, such as the thoracic or abdominal cavities. Patient factors requiring a general anesthetic may include age, mental or emotional state, or individual preference.

Monitoring

All vital functions of the patient receiving a general anesthetic are continuously monitored. Heart rate and EKG, blood pressure, respirations, oxygen saturation, expired gases (**end-tidal CO_2**), and temperature are closely observed to assess the physiologic condition of the patient. Some surgical procedures also require monitoring of urinary output; others require more intensive cardiovascular monitoring using devices such as a pulmonary artery catheter.

Phases

There are five phases of general anesthesia: preinduction, induction, maintenance, emergence, and recovery (Table 13–3). The preinduction phase includes preoperative assessment and preparation of the patient, both physically and psychologically (see Chapter 12). The intraoperative phases of general anesthesia are induction, maintenance, and emergence. Recovery is the postoperative phase.

The induction phase begins in the operating room. Here, the patient is preoxygenated and medications are given to initiate a general anesthetic. Induction agents are administered, usually followed by a muscle relaxant. During general anesthesia, the patient's respirations are controlled with ventilation. Drugs used to paralyze the surgical field also affect the respiratory muscles, so the patient's respirations must be controlled by ventilation. Under direct visualization with a **laryngoscope** (Fig. 13–9), an **endotracheal tube** is placed through the patient's vocal cords into the trachea. This process is called **intubation.** The circulator usually assists the anesthesia provider during this procedure, often applying cricoid pressure as needed (Fig. 13–10). Cricoid pressure is used to gently compress the esophagus, reducing risk of aspiration. The endotracheal tube is connected to a ventilator (Fig. 13–11) to control respirations.

Alternatively, the airway may be managed with a laryngeal masked airway or LMA (Fig. 13–12). The LMA is a reusable, autoclavable airway used when an endotracheal tube is not required. After induction of anesthesia, an LMA is inserted, the cuff inflated and connected to the ventilator. The LMA, which does not require laryngoscopy or muscle relaxation, is particularly useful for ambulatory surgical procedures. Contraindications include obesity, hiatal hernia, history of gastroesophageal reflux disease (GERD), low pulmonary compliance, or the absence of adequate NPO status.

The maintenance phase begins after intubation or airway insertion, and continues until the surgical procedure has been completed. As the procedure is completed, the emergence phase begins, during which the anesthetic agents are discontinued and allowed to wear off. In some cases, the anesthetic agents

Table 13-3 **Phases of a General Anesthetic Course**

Preinduction
Induction
Maintenance
Emergence
Recovery

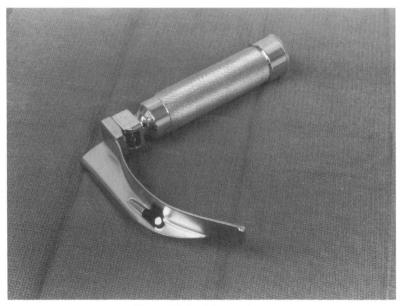

Figure 13-9   A laryngoscope.

may be reversed to permit the patient to gradually awaken. When the patient is breathing on his or her own, the endotracheal tube is removed, a process called **extubation.** If all vital signs are stable, the patient is carefully moved to a trans-

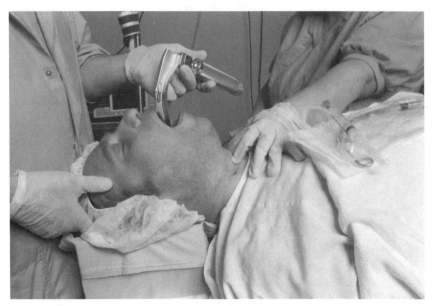

Figure 13-10   Application of cricoid pressure prior to endotracheal intubation.

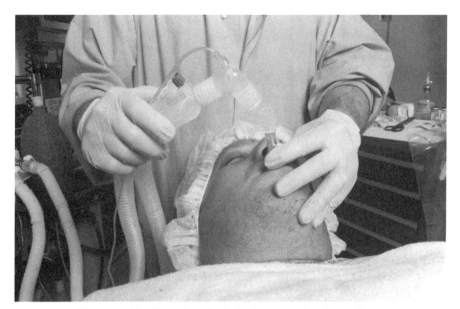

Figure 13-11   The endotracheal tube is connected to the ventilator.

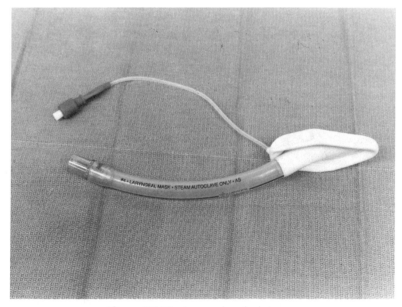

Figure 13-12   Laryngeal masked airway.

port stretcher and taken to the postanesthesia care unit (PACU) for the recovery phase. The anesthesia provider gives a detailed report to the PACU staff nurses who will closely monitor the patient during the recovery phase.

☞ Of special importance to the surgical team is the fact that the patient may experience a period of agitation or excitement during both induction and emergence. The effect of loud noises may be intensified during this time, inducing a stress reaction in the patient. Thus, the surgical technologist and all members of the surgical team must minimize unnecessary operating room noise during these phases.

Components

Administration of a general anesthetic includes four major components: **narcosis** (stupor), **analgesia** (painlessness), **amnesia** (memory impairment), and muscle relaxation (Table 13–4). That is, the patient must remain asleep, pain-free, and flaccid while retaining no explicit memory of the event. Many different agents are used to accomplish these required components. As the individual agents are discussed, their actions will be described within the three intraoperative phases of a general anesthetic.

Methods

Two methods, or routes, are used to administer general anesthetic agents: inhalation and intravenous injection. An inhalation anesthetic is administered as a gas the patient breathes while intravenous agents are administered directly into the bloodstream through a small catheter placed in a vein. The term *balanced anesthesia* refers to the technique which uses a combination of inhalation and intravenous agents.

Another anesthesia technique uses a combination of a regional block, such as epidural or spinal, and a light general anesthetic. This technique is useful for major vascular procedures because it decreases the amount of general anesthetic agents required, and provides effective postoperative pain control.

Table 13-4 **Components of General Anesthesia**

Amnesia
Analgesia
Narcosis
Muscle Relaxation

Agents

Several different classes of drugs have been used to achieve general anesthesia. Multiple agents are used to provide narcosis, analgesia, amnesia, and muscle relaxation. These drugs will be discussed in the phases of general anesthesia in which they are administered. The broad categories covered are intravenous induction agents, narcotics, inhalation agents, neuromuscular blocking agents, and emergence agents.

INTRAVENOUS INDUCTION AGENTS

The most common intravenous induction agents are either barbiturates or benzodiazepines. There are also individual agents, such as ketamine, etomidate, and propofol.

Barbiturates are ultra–short-acting induction agents derived from barbituric acid. The most frequently used barbiturates are thiopental (Pentothal) and methohexital (Brevital). Thiopental, for instance, takes just 15 seconds to travel from the injection site to the brain; thus it is rapidly taken up by the brain, but it is also rapidly eliminated. Barbiturates induce anesthesia, but they have no analgesic effect; patients may therefore be agitated and disoriented during the emergence phase because of the pain they begin to feel.

Benzodiazepines, which have both sedative and amnesiac effects, are used both preoperatively and as induction agents. The most common benzodiazepine used in surgery is midazolam (Versed). Others include diazepam (Valium) and lorazepam (Ativan), which are often used preoperatively; however, they are rarely used as induction agents because of slower onset and longer elimination time. Benzodiazepines rapidly penetrate the blood–brain barrier, producing a loss of consciousness in 45–90 seconds. Like barbiturates, benzodiazepines provide no analgesia.

Ketamine (Ketalar) is a dissociative agent used for induction and maintenance of general anesthesia. Chemically related to the drug PCP (phencyclidine or "angel dust"), ketamine is a powerful analgesic and amnesiac whose onset of action is 30–60 seconds after intravenous injection. When ketamine is used, patients appear to be awake and their eyes may be open; however, they are dissociated from their environment and they are amnestic. Ketamine can cause hallucinations and involuntary movements, making patients difficult to handle. It also exaggerates the effect of sudden loud noises. Ketamine is most often utilized for superficial procedures of short duration, such as painful dressing changes, debridements, or skin grafts. Ketamine does not produce any skeletal muscle relaxation.

Etomidate (Amidate) produces an unconscious state in less than a minute, but provides no analgesia and no muscle relaxation. This agent is often used for patients with compromised heart function who cannot tolerate the drop in blood pressure often seen with other induction agents. Etomidate is ideal for brief procedures such as cardioversion. It is also useful for induction in trauma patients, who may be **hypovolemic** and hence unable to tolerate any additional hypotension.

Propofol (Diprivan) is chemically unrelated to any other anesthetic agent. It is a sedative/hypnotic which is injected intravenously in doses of 2–2.5 mg/kg. Propofol produces an unconscious state within a minute. Because of its brief duration, patients recover alert and free of the usual side effects of an anesthetic agent. Propofol provides poor analgesia and no muscle relaxation. Among the inactive components of the propofol emulsion are soybean oil, glycerol, and egg lecithin; thus, propofol is contraindicated in patients with a known allergy to eggs. Propofol has a characteristic milky white appearance (Fig. 13–13). Strict aseptic technique must be maintained when handling propofol because it contains no antimicrobial preservatives and can support rapid growth of microorganisms. Potential adverse effects include bradycardia, hypotension, and apnea. Some patients report a stinging sensation at the injection site.

NARCOTICS

Narcotics are often given during maintenance of general anesthesia because of their analgesic effects, which may reduce the amount of anesthetic agents

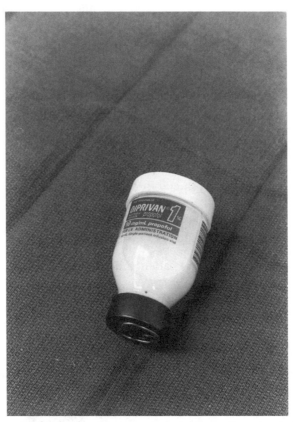

Figure 13-13 Propofol (Diprivan) is an intravenous induction agent. (Reproduced with permission of Zeneca Pharmaceuticals, Wilmington, DE.)

needed. In extremely high doses, narcotics can be used to induce stupor. Narcotics such as fentanyl (Sublimaze), alfentanil (Alfenta), and sufentanil (Sufenta) are frequently used during general anesthesia. Fentanyl, alfentanil, and sufentanil are called synthetic narcotics because they resemble morphine pharmacologically, but are not naturally occurring. These drugs are useful in anesthesia because of their relatively short action and intense analgesic effect. Synthetic narcotics are more potent analgesics than morphine; but, at equivalent analgesic doses, they cause the same degree of respiratory depression.

Fentanyl is 100 times more potent than morphine. This drug has a rapid onset, about 30 seconds, with a duration of 45–60 minutes. Fentanyl provides analgesia plus some sedation. When used as the sole anesthetic agent, the dose for induction is 5–30 mcg/kg of body weight. When used in addition to other agents, the dose is 1–10 mcg/kg. Alfentanil has one-fourth the potency of fentanyl; it has a slower onset, about 1–2 minutes, and lasts just 10–15 minutes. Alfentanil is classified as an ultra–short-acting narcotic. When used as a sole anesthetic agent, the induction dosage is 50–150 mcg/kg. When used in combination with other agents, the dose is 10–25 mcg/kg. Sufentanil is 5–10 times more potent than fentanyl; but it is more rapidly cleared from the body, providing a very rapid recovery. Onset is immediate, with effects lasting 20–45 minutes. When used as a sole anesthetic agent, the induction dose is 2–10 mcg/kg. If used with other agents, the dose is .2–.6 mcg/kg. See Table 13–5 for a comparison of narcotics used for maintenance of general anesthesia.

INHALATION INDUCTION AND MAINTENANCE AGENTS

The first inhalation anesthetics used were ether, chloroform, nitrous oxide, and cyclopropane. Of these, only nitrous oxide is in use currently. While ether and cyclopropane are explosive, chloroform is toxic to the liver. Halothane (Fluothane), introduced in 1956, was the first nonexplosive inhalation agent developed.

Inhalation agents are relatively easy to administer, control, and assess and are eliminated from the body quickly, most via the pulmonary, hepatic, and renal systems. Inhalation agents, which are measured by the percentage of vapor present in the mixture the patient inhales (Fig. 13–14), diffuse into the blood from the

Table 13-5 Comparison of Narcotics Used for Maintenance of General Anesthesia

Generic Name	Trade Name	Dose (mcg/kg)	Onset	Duration (minutes)
Fentanyl	Sublimaze	1–10	30 sec	45–60
Alfentanil	Alfenta	10–25	1–2 min	10–15
Sufentanil	Sufenta	.2–.6	immediate	20–45

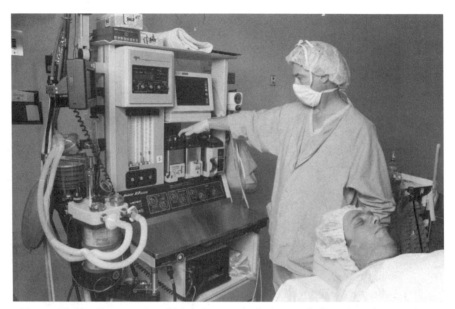

Figure 13-14 Concentration of inhalation anesthetics is controlled in an anesthesia machine.

air in the alveoli, then rapidly diffuse out of the blood and into the brain—the site of action. Several inhalation agents are routinely used in surgery, each will be briefly discussed. The disadvantages of inhalation agents include an increased potential for cardiovascular depression and lack of postoperative analgesia.

Nitrous oxide (N_2O)—a colorless, odorless, tasteless gas—is the most widely used inhalation anesthetic in clinical practice. Nitrous oxide provides rapid onset and emergence and is completely eliminated by the lungs. Its mild analgesic and amnesiac characteristics make it an excellent adjunct to volatile liquid agents. Nitrous oxide is often used in conjunction with volatile liquid agents in order to reduce the amount of the latter needed. A common mixture of inhalation agents might be 56–70% N_2O, 30–35% O_2, and .5–2% halothane, enflurane, or isoflurane. A muscle relaxant must also be given if needed.

Halothane (Fluothane) is a volatile liquid agent frequently used for pediatric patients because it reaches desired alveolar concentrations quite rapidly in children. Halothane is contraindicated for Cesarean section because it relaxes smooth muscle; thus, the uterus may not contract as needed to control postpartum bleeding. Halothane can sensitize the heart to agents like epinephrine, thus causing arrhythmias. Consequently, the surgical technologist should keep accurate measurements of any epinephrine used from the sterile field. About 70–80% of halothane is eliminated by the lungs and the remainder is metabolized by the liver. A side effect associated with halothane administration is hepatic dysfunction, commonly seen in middle-aged obese women.

Two inhalation agents—enflurane (Ethrane) and isoflurane (Forane)—are closely related to halothane in action, but are more rapid in onset and are more effectively eliminated from the body by the lungs. Newer inhalation agents, such as desflurane (Suprane) and sevoflurane (Sevoflurane), are quite similar to the other volatile liquids, except that they provide more precise control of maintenance and more rapid induction and emergence. See Table 13–6 for a list of inhalation anesthetic agents.

☞ Inhalation anesthetic agents (except for nitrous oxide), either alone or in combination with succinylcholine, have been identified as triggering agents of a rare but life-threatening condition called malignant hyperthermia (see Chapter 15).

NEUROMUSCULAR BLOCKING AGENTS

Patients under general anesthesia may be asleep, pain-free, and memory-free, but their skeletal muscles will continue to respond to stimuli. In order to receive an endotracheal tube, the patient must be adequately paralyzed; i.e., their muscles must be relaxed. And during the surgical procedure, the patient's muscles must be paralyzed to better expose the surgical site, especially in the abdomen. (See Insight 13–2.)

Muscle Physiology Review

There are three types of muscle tissue: cardiac, smooth, and skeletal. Muscles function in circulation, labor and delivery, and intestinal movements, as well as in body movement. In order for a muscle to contract, it must be stimulated by a motor nerve. The neuromuscular junction is an area where the motor nerve axon is very near the muscle fiber. The space between an axon and a muscle fiber is called a synapse. When a neurotransmitter called acetylcholine (ACh) is released from the axon, it leaps across the synapse and binds to receptor sites on the surface of the muscle fiber (the sarcolemma). Acetylcholine causes an impulse to spread across the muscle fiber to the sarcoplasmic reticulum, releasing calcium

Table 13-6 Inhalation Anesthetics

Generic Name	Trade Name
Gas	
Nitrous oxide (N_2O)	
Volatile liquid (vapor)	
Halothane	Fluothane
Enflurane	Ethrane
Isoflurane	Forane
Desflurane	Suprane
Sevoflurane	Sevoflurane

INSIGHT 13–2 | THE FIRST MUSCLE RELAXANT

The earliest known muscle relaxant was curare. It is a toxin that is extracted from plants found in the rainforest. Indigenous peoples on three separate continents—South America, Africa, and Southeast Asia—used curare on the tips of darts to immobilize monkeys and other tree-dwelling animals. Once discovered by western culture, curare was used in the experimental laboratory for various purposes. A German report in 1912 described the use of curare on humans as an adjunct to anesthesia; however, the report was generally ignored. It wasn't until 1942 that curare was first used in surgery to relax abdominal muscles of a patient undergoing an appendectomy. Discovery of the benefits of curare radically changed anesthesia practice. Patients could now be routinely intubated, a sporadic practice prior to the use of curare. Since curare, many agents have been developed to provide muscle relaxation.

ions from storage. Calcium ions alter muscle filaments, exposing myosin-binding sites; this results in muscle contraction, known as depolarization. Repolarization is the process of muscle fiber relaxation, i.e., returning to a resting state. For muscle fibers to return to a resting state, ACh must disconnect from the receptor sites and be broken down, or recycled, by an enzyme called acetylcholinesterase. This enzyme, which is present on the sarcolemma, breaks down ACh and terminates the contraction. Calcium ions are then transported back into the sarcoplasmic reticulum for storage and later release. Depolarizing muscle relaxants act like ACh; they bind with receptor sites and initiate a contraction (depolarization). Such contractions are observed as **fasciculations.** Subsequent contractions are prevented as long as the depolarizing muscle relaxant stays on the binding sites. Nondepolarizing muscle relaxants are ACh antagonists; they block receptor sites and prevent ACh binding, thus preventing a contraction.

☞ Students should consult an anatomy and physiology text to review the physiology of muscle contraction in more depth.

There are two basic types of muscle relaxants classified according to their action on the motor end-plate: depolarizing and nondepolarizing (Fig. 13–15). Examples of each type will be listed with a brief description.

Succinylcholine (Anectine) is the only depolarizing muscle relaxant in use today. Succinylcholine acts similarly to the neurotransmitter acetylcholine (ACh), but its duration is longer. It causes persistent depolarization (sustained contraction) and produces fasciculations followed by **flaccidity.** Succinylcholine acts rapidly, and its effects are seen in 30–60 seconds. Duration of effects is also short, usually only 4–6 minutes; but because no antagonist or reversal agent is currently available, succinylcholine must be allowed to wear off. Problems have been associated with administration of succinylcholine. These include increased intracranial pressure, increased intragastric pressure (which increases the potential for

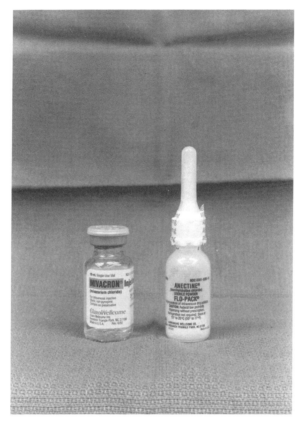

Figure 13-15 Muscle relaxants. (Reproduced with permission of Glaxo Wellcome, Inc.)

regurgitation), and muscle soreness postoperatively. Elevated serum potassium levels have been noted in burn patients receiving succinylcholine. Patients with pseudocholinesterase deficiency may experience prolonged respiratory paralysis because succinylcholine is not eliminated effectively without that enzyme.

☞ Succinylcholine has been identified as a triggering agent for malignant hyperthermia. See Chapter 15 for additional information.

There are several nondepolarizing muscle relaxants. These include atracurium besylate (Tracrium), mivacurium chloride (Mivacron), pancuronium bromide (Pavulon), rocuronium bromide (Zemuron), tubocurarine chloride (Curare), and vecuronium bromide (Norcuron). Nondepolarizing muscle relaxants prevent muscle contractions by binding to cholinergic receptors, preventing the uptake of acetylcholine. Nondepolarizing muscle relaxants do not cause fasciculations and may be used prior to administration of succinylcholine to prevent fasciculations. The selection of a particular nondepolarizing muscle relaxant depends on its pharmacologic properties, such as onset and duration of effects, and side effects, such as those seen in the cardiovascular system. See Table 13–7 for a comparison of neuromuscular blocking agents. Adverse effects of nondepolarizing muscle relaxants on the cardiovascular system include hypotension or hypertension, tachycardia, bradycardia, and arrhythmias. Dosage is variable, depending upon onset time and depth of block required. Nondepolarizing muscle relaxants may be reversed if necessary with an antagonist such as neostigmine (Prostigmine). Neostigmine works by competing with acetylcholine for attachment to acetylcholinesterase. This competition causes a buildup of acetylcholine, which facilitates transmission of impulses across the neuromuscular junction.

EMERGENCE AGENTS

The emergence phase of anesthesia is quite variable, depending on the anesthetic agents used and the individual patient. Few medications are given during emergence; however, some reversal agents may be administered just prior to emergence. Naloxone (Narcan) will reverse a narcotic. Benzodiazepines may be reversed with flumazenil (Mazicon). If necessary, nondepolarizing muscle relaxants may be reversed with neostigmine (Prostigmin).

☞ The surgical patient may experience an excitement period during emergence, which can be greatly affected by noise and activity. The surgical technologist and all team members must be aware that sudden, loud noise during emergence may cause severe adverse reactions in the surgical patient.

Table 13-7 Comparison of Neuromuscular Blocking Agents

Agent	Duration (min)	CVS Effects	Excretion
Succinylcholine (Anectine)	4–6	Hypotension Hypertension Bradycardia Tachycardia Arrhythmias	Plasma pseudocholinesterase
Atracurium besylate (Tracrium)	20–35	Hypotension Vasodilation Bradycardia Tachycardia	Hepatic Renal
Mivacurium chloride (Mivacron)	6–10	Hypotension Vasodilation Bradycardia Tachycardia	Plasma cholinesterase
Pancuronium bromide (Pavulon)	40–65	Tachycardia Hypertension	Renal Hepatic
Rocuronium bromide (Zemuron)	15–85	Arrhythmias Tachycardia	Hepatic Renal
Vecuronium bromide (Norcuron)	25–30	Bradycardia	Hepatic Renal

Upon emergence, the patient may be extubated and transferred to a transport stretcher. Occasionally, the patient must remain intubated and will be transported to the postanesthesia care unit (PACU) with ventilation via an ambu bag. The circulator will accompany the patient and the anesthesia provider to PACU for recovery.

Summary

Accomplishing anesthesia is an art as well as a science. Various drugs and techniques have been utilized to achieve a state of anesthesia. While theories abound, the exact mechanism of action of anesthetic drugs remains unknown.

Three main types of anesthesia are available today: local (with or without MAC), regional blockade, and general. If a local or regional block is administered, the patient will remain conscious, yet will be pain-free. Several agents are used to produce local and regional anesthesia, and there are many applications for these techniques.

In some cases, it is important that the patient be under general anesthesia, i.e., unconscious, pain-free, and immobile. General anesthesia may be necessary due to patient factors or the nature of the surgical procedure.

There are five phases of administration of a general anesthetic: preinduction, induction, maintenance, emergence, and recovery. Four major components must be accomplished in general anesthesia: narcosis, analgesia, amnesia, and muscle relaxation. The two methods or routes used to deliver general anesthetics are intravenous and inhalation. Intravenous induction agents include barbiturates, benzodiazepines, ketamine, etomidate, and propofol. Narcotics administered as an adjunct to general anesthesia are fentanyl, alfentanil, and sufentanil. Common inhalation agents include the gas nitrous oxide as well as many volatile liquid anesthetics such as halothane. Muscle relaxants, given as an adjunct to general anesthesia, are categorized as depolarizing and nondepolarizing neuromuscular blockers. Agents that may be administered during emergence include naloxone, flumazenil, and neostigmine.

Anesthesia is a complex physiologic state, often taken for granted by operating room personnel. The surgical technologist must understand the basic concepts of anesthesia, as well as the names of common agents used in order to function effectively on the surgical team.

REVIEW

1. What does the term *anesthesia* mean?

2. What are the three major types of anesthesia?

3. What kinds of surgical procedures may be performed under each type of anesthesia?

4. Which agents are used to provide local and regional anesthesia?

5. How is local anesthesia like MAC? How are the two types different?

6. Can you list some types of regional blocks? What kinds of procedures may be performed under each?

7. What is the scrubbed surgical technologist doing during each phase of a general anesthetic? What is the circulating surgical technologist doing during each phase?

8. What are the four components of a general anesthetic?

9. What two routes are used to deliver general anesthesia?

10. Can you list common agents used in each phase of general anesthesia?

11. Match generic and trade names of drugs used in anesthesia.

___fentanyl   a. Anectine
___halothane   b. Fluothane
___lidocaine   c. Sublimaze
___succinylcholine   d. Xylocaine

12. How do muscle relaxants work?

13. How are depolarizing and nondepolarizing muscle relaxants alike? How are they different?

CHAPTER 14

Blood and Fluid Replacement

OBJECTIVES

Upon completion of this chapter you should be able to:

1 List basic functions of the blood.
2 State average adult circulating volume of blood.
3 Describe patients who may need blood replacement.
4 List the formed elements present in blood.
5 Define terms and abbreviations related to blood and fluid replacement.
6 State normal range of hemoglobin and hematocrit.
7 List major blood types.
8 Briefly describe antigen/antibody interactions in blood types.
9 State indications for blood replacement in the surgical patient.
10 List available options for blood replacement.

11 Describe components of whole blood used for replacement.
12 Describe the process of intraoperative autotransfusion.
13 List blood substitutes used in surgery.
14 Describe the procedure for blood replacement in surgery using donor blood.
15 Briefly describe the physiology of fluid loss in the surgical patient.
16 List three fluid electrolytes crucial to homeostasis.
17 List three functions of electrolytes in homeostasis.
18 State three objectives of parenteral fluid therapy in surgery.
19 List common IV fluids and their purposes in surgery.
20 List supplies needed to start an intravenous line.

KEY TERMS

Antibody A protein that reacts with a specific antigen.

Antigen A protein marker on the surface of cells.

Arrhythmia Variation from the normal rhythm of the heartbeat.

Autologous Related to self; belonging to the same organism.

Autotransfusion Reinfusion of a patient's own blood.

Electrolyte Chemical substance that dissociates into electrically charged particles when dissolved in water.

Hematocrit The volume of red blood cells in a volume of whole blood, expressed as a percentage.

Hemoglobin A protein found in red blood cells that transports molecular oxygen in the blood.

Hyperkalemia Abnormally high potassium concentration in the blood.

Hypokalemia Abnormally low potassium concentration in the blood.

Hypovolemia Abnormally low volume of circulating fluid (plasma) in the body.

Isotonic Exhibiting equal osmotic pressure; pertains to solutions in which body cells can be bathed without net flow of water across the semipermeable cell membrane. (Isotonic solutions do not cause hemolysis.)

Metabolic acidosis A pathologic condition resulting from accumulation of acid in the blood or body tissues.

Phagocytosis Engulfing of microorganisms or other cells and foreign particles by white blood cells (phagocytes).

One of the primary goals of surgical patient care is to maintain the patient in as stable a physiologic state as possible. Blood and fluid replacement are two of the most common means used in surgery to assist in maintaining homeostasis. Blood loss may be due to trauma or to the surgical procedure itself. The volume of blood lost must be carefully assessed and replaced if significant. The surgical patient's fluid and electrolyte balance must also be assessed and monitored.

Most surgical patients will have had nothing to eat or drink in the eight hours prior to surgery, so fluid replacement is usually indicated. The surgical technologist will assist with blood or fluid replacement procedures in the operating room daily.

Blood Replacement

Physiology Review

Blood performs several critical functions in maintaining homeostasis. It is used to transport oxygen, nutrients, wastes, hormones and enzymes throughout the body. Blood also maintains the body's acid–base balance (pH), its temperature, and its water content. The immune response is carried through the circulatory system as well. Blood is so crucial to maintaining life processes that it has a self-protection mechanism—clotting—to prevent harmful loss.

In an average adult, the circulating blood volume is approximately 70 mL/kg of body mass. In order to keep the body functioning normally, this blood volume should be maintained. Some surgical patients are at high risk for substantial blood loss during surgery; these include patients needing cardiac and peripheral vascular procedures, or those with trauma. The goal of blood replacement in scheduled surgical procedures is to maintain the circulating volume of blood as well as its oxygen-carrying capacity.

Blood consists of two main components: formed elements and plasma (fluid). The formed elements include erythrocytes (red blood cells, RBCs), leukocytes (white blood cells, WBCs), and platelets. Erythrocytes contain **hemoglobin,** a protein responsible for transport of oxygen and carbon dioxide between the lungs and the cells. Leukocytes provide protection against foreign microbes by **phagocytosis** and antibody production. Platelets mediate the clotting process.

Most surgical patients undergo laboratory tests to determine the amount of hemoglobin (Hgb) present in their blood. A normal hemoglobin level is 12–16 g/100 mL of blood in adult females and 14–18 g/100 mL in adult males. A low hemoglobin level indicates reduced oxygen-carrying capacity. Since oxygen levels must be optimum during general anesthesia, elective surgery may be canceled if the hemoglobin dips below normal levels. Another important measure of the oxygen-carrying capacity of the blood is **hematocrit.** Hematocrit is the volume of erythrocytes in a given volume of blood and is expressed as a percentage. Normal hematocrit levels range from 35 to 50%, varying by age and sex (Table 14–1).

In cases of known or anticipated blood loss, the patient's blood must be typed and cross-matched in order to administer compatible donor blood. The blood type is determined by proteins called **antigens** present on the surface of RBCs. Blood type is inherited, and there are many types and groupings based on the antigens present on the RBCs. The major groupings of concern in surgery are ABO and Rh. Patients may be type A, B, AB, or O. Type A blood contains the A

Table 14–1 **Hemoglobin and Hematocrit Values**

	Females	Males
Hemoglobin	12–16 g/100 mL	14–18 g/100 mL
Hematocrit	37–47%	40–54%

antigen, type B has the B antigen, type AB contains both, and type O blood has neither. Blood is also designated as Rh-positive (Rh antigen present) or Rh-negative (no Rh antigen present). Each person also has the corresponding **antibody** present in his or her plasma; i.e., type A has anti-B, type B has anti-A, type O has both anti-A and anti-B, and type AB has neither (Fig. 14–1). If type A blood is

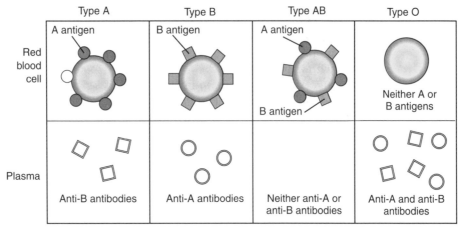

A

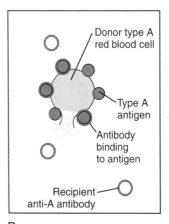

B

Figure 14–1 Antigen and antibody in blood types.

administered to a type B patient, the recipient's antibodies will attack the donor RBCs, causing a potentially fatal transfusion reaction. A blood cross-match is performed to determine compatibility between the donor and the recipient. A sample of donor RBCs is mixed with the recipient's serum and the results are examined to determine compatibility. For further explanation of the physiology of blood, please refer to your anatomy and physiology textbook.

Indications for Blood Replacement

The first recorded blood transfusion occurred in 1667 when a 15–year-old male was given lamb's blood. This method was popular for a time until transfusion reactions were recognized and reported. Since the discovery that even all human blood is not alike, many advances have been made in blood transfusion therapy. Today, blood transfusions are routine.

The most common indication for blood replacement in surgery is **hypovolemia** or circulatory shock, seen most frequently in trauma and vascular procedures. Other indications include restoration of the oxygen-carrying capacity as seen in anemic patients, and to maintain clotting properties as needed in patients with hemophilia.

Trauma patients may be in critical need of blood in order to sustain vital functions. If immediate replacement is required, and the patient's blood type is known, type-specific–only RBCs (packed cells) may be administered along with fluid volume support. If the patient's blood type is unknown, O-negative blood may be administered. In either case, the surgeon must document the need for blood release without compatibility testing.

Options for Blood Replacement

There are several options available to replace blood loss in surgery; these include use of donor blood, **autologous** donation, **autotransfusion,** or use of blood substitutes. Each blood replacement option has indications, advantages, and disadvantages. Some of these options may not be feasible in certain cases, depending on the situation.

DONOR BLOOD

A common method of blood replacement is the use of donor blood. A blood bank is responsible for collecting, processing and releasing donor blood for use. Donor blood, while carefully tested, does present some risk for transmission of blood-borne pathogens and is used only when clearly indicated.

Blood is separated during processing into components and then administered to treat specific needs. Component replacement therapy is an effective and efficient use of limited resources because a unit of donor whole blood, separated into components, can be used to treat several patients.

Whole Blood

Whole blood consisting of formed elements plus plasma is rarely used for transfusion today. Whole, fresh blood is indicated only in cases of acute, massive blood loss.

Packed Cells (RBCs)

Most transfusions of donor blood in surgery involve the use of packed red blood cells (RBCs). The use of packed RBCs with a synthetic volume expander has proven to be as effective as whole blood, while reducing the risks of whole blood transfusion reactions. Packed cells are obtained by removing approximately 200 mL of plasma from 1 unit (500 mL) of whole blood. The infusion of RBCs helps restore the oxygen-carrying capacity of the patient's own circulatory system. Intravenous fluids are administered concurrently to restore circulating volume.

Plasma

Plasma may be administered when clotting factors are needed in addition to circulating volume. This need is frequently seen when several units of blood have been replaced, as the clotting factors have been removed from donor blood. Plasma is not used for volume expansion alone, because albumin and synthetic expanders are as effective and eliminate the risk of transmission of blood-borne diseases. Plasma is stored as fresh-frozen plasma (FFP) to preserve clotting factors and thawed in a water bath prior to use. It must be administered type-specific and used within 6 hours of thawing.

Platelets

Platelets are administered in surgery when large amounts of donor blood have been used to replace the patient's volume. Because the platelets have been removed from donor blood, the result of massive transfusions may be an inability of the patient's circulatory system to clot properly. Platelets are infused to restore a more normal clotting process. At room temperature, platelets must be continually gently agitated to prevent clumping.

Cryoprecipitate

Cryoprecipitate is a concentration of clotting factor VIII, which is used to treat hemophilia A. Cryoprecipitate may be administered in surgery when massive amounts of blood have been replaced, severely impacting the normal coagulation process.

AUTOLOGOUS DONATION

Patients scheduled for elective surgical procedures in which blood loss is anticipated, such as a total hip replacement, may be allowed to donate their own blood prior to surgery. This process is called autologous transfusion and usually involves two units of blood. Most patients can safely donate two units of whole blood over a period of weeks just prior to their scheduled procedure, possibly eliminating the need for donor blood. The patient's blood is collected, processed, stored, and released for surgery by the blood bank. Patients often choose this option, if available, to protect themselves from potential blood-borne disease transmission.

AUTOTRANSFUSION

Another form of autologous donation used intraoperatively and postoperatively is called autotransfusion. Autotransfusion involves the collection, processing, and return of the patient's own blood during the surgical procedure using "cell-saver" technology (Fig. 14–2). Autotransfusion is routinely used during open-

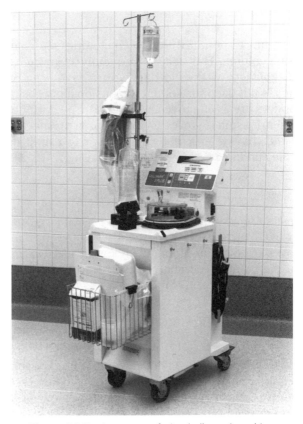

Figure 14–2 An autotransfusion (cell-saver) machine.

heart surgery, peripheral vascular procedures, and some trauma procedures such as splenectomy. Autotransfusion has several advantages over the use of donor blood, including immediate replacement of blood loss without the potential for transfusion reaction or delay for blood typing and cross-matching and no risk of transmission of blood-borne pathogens. In addition, patients with religious objections to donated blood often do not object to autotransfusion. Autotransfusion is not suitable for all patients, as some trauma patients may have lost so much blood already that there is little volume left to salvage. A disadvantage of autotransfusion is that it cannot be used in the presence of cancer cells, infection, or gross contamination, e.g., open gastrointestinal tract. Autotransfusion is generally contraindicated during cesarean section due to the presence of amniotic fluid. Autotransfusion is commonplace in most operating rooms today and is an effective option for replacement of blood lost during certain surgical procedures.

BLOOD SUBSTITUTES

When donated blood or autotransfusion is not immediately available for emergency procedures, blood substitutes may be used to temporarily maintain a circulating volume. As soon as possible, packed RBCs will be administered to restore the oxygen-carrying capacity of the patient's blood. There are several blood substitutes available.

Albumin is available in concentrations of 5% or 25% in sodium chloride solution. Albumin is most frequently used in the treatment of hypovolemic shock, as seen in burn patients who have lost fluid volume but not RBCs.

Dextran is a plasma volume expander used to treat hypovolemic shock. It is packaged for IV administration, 6% Dextran 70 in .9% sodium chloride (Macrodex) or 10% Dextran 40 in 5% dextrose or .9% sodium chloride (Rheomacrodex). The usual dose is 500 mL.

Hetastarch (Hespan), which is also used as a volume expander, is made from cornstarch. Hetastarch comes in a 6% solution in .9% sodium chloride.

Procedure for Donor Blood Replacement in Surgery

The process for administration of donated blood products must be carefully monitored at each step to prevent transfusion of incompatible elements. Transfusion of incompatible blood or blood products can cause a fatal transfusion reaction. The patient who needs a transfusion will be typed and cross-matched and identified with a special wrist band. A requisition slip (Fig. 14–3) with multiple carbon copies will be sent to the blood bank with patient name, identification number, amount and type of blood ordered. A copy of the requisition is sent back to surgery with each unit of released blood. Meticulous records are kept in the blood bank on each unit, and the transporter will be required to verify correct information with blood bank personnel and sign out each unit released.

BLOOD BANK REQUISITION

REGIONAL MEDICAL CENTER
ANYTOWN, USA

☐ PACKED CELLS ☐ FRESH FROZEN PLASMA ☐ PLATELETS SINGLE DONOR ☐ PLATELETS RANDOM | OTHER (SPECIFY)

UNIT NO. ABO & Rh	PATIENT NO. ABO & Rh	EXPIRATION DATE
		X-MATCHED BY-DATE ☐ COMPATIBLE

DATE ____________

PATIENT ____________ BIRTH DATE ____________

PHYSCIAN ____________

HOSPITAL NO. ____________

BLOOD BANK RELEASE	TRANSFUSION STARTING RECORD		TRANSFUSION CHECK LIST
DATE BLOOD TAKEN/TECH	TRANSFUSION ORDERED BY	TRANSFUSION STARTED DATE	☐ Order verified from chart ☐ Verbal Order ☐ I have established the identity of the patient.
TIME TAKEN A.M. P.M.	I HAVE CAREFULLY COMPLETED THE CHECK LIST AND ATTACHED PART 1 TO PATIENT'S CHART	TRANSFUSION STARTED TIME A.M. P.M.	☐ The patient's name and hospital number agree with those on the tag. ☐ The blood type and Rh on the tag agree with those on the unit.
TAKEN BY	SIGNED* MD RN		☐ Blood unit number marked on the tag agrees with the number on the unit. ☐ The blood is not outdated.
	*MUST BE SIGNED BY PERSON STARTING TRANSFUSION		

Figure 14–3 Sample blood requisition slip.

Once the donor units reach the surgical suite, they are to be placed in an appropriate blood refrigerator, which must have continuous temperature monitoring. Any units needed for immediate transfusion will be taken directly to the operating room. Both circulator and anesthesia provider will verify the patient and donor unit information prior to administration.

When multiple units of blood are to be administered over a short period of time, the blood must be warmed to prevent hypothermia. Several types of blood warmers are available (Fig. 14–4). Because minute pieces of debris are present in processed blood, microfilters will be used to reduce the risk of post-transfusion complications. If blood must be transfused rapidly, a blood pump will be used. Different types of blood pumps are available, from simple pneumatic pumps to complex electric or battery-operated units that calibrate the infusion rate precisely.

Fluid and Electrolyte Management in Surgery

Physiology Review

Body fluid contains two major types of solutes, **electrolytes** (ionic compounds) and nonelectrolytes (nonionic compounds). The major electrolytes break down into sodium (Na^+), chloride (Cl^-), potassium (K^+), calcium (Ca^{2+}), phosphate (HPO_4^{2-}), and magnesium (Mg^{2+}) ions. Other electrolytes are bicarbonate (HCO_3^-), sulfate (SO_4^{2-}), and carbonic acid (H_2CO_3). The nonelectrolytes present in normal body fluid are glucose, urea, and creatinine. Electrolytes have three main pur-

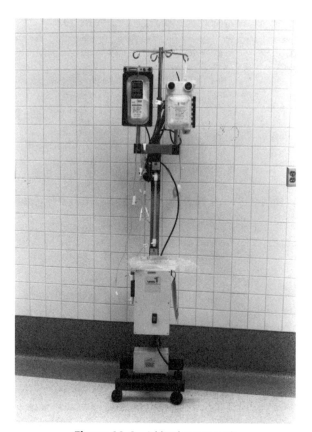

Figure 14–4   A blood warmer unit.

poses in homeostasis: controlling the volume of body water by osmotic pressure, maintaining the acid–base balance, and serving as essential minerals. See Table 14–2 for a list of major electrolytes and functions.

Calcium is necessary for the formation and function of bones and teeth. Calcium is also involved in the blood-clotting process, neurotransmitter release, muscle contraction, and cardiac function. Chloride helps regulate osmotic pressure between intracellular and extracellular spaces. Magnesium plays an important part in the sodium–potassium pump and also activates enzymes required to break down adenosine triphosphate (ATP). Phosphate is stored in teeth and bone and is released when needed. Phosphate is a necessary element in the formation of DNA and RNA, in synthesis of ATP, and in buffering of acid–base reactions.

Potassium (K^+) serves several critical functions in homeostasis. Potassium helps maintain fluid volume in cells, controls pH, and is vital in the transmission of nerve impulses. Either too much potassium, **hyperkalemia,** or too little, **hypokalemia,** causes serious metabolic problems. Since potassium is critical to

Table 14–2 Major Electrolytes and Functions

Electrolyte	Chemical Symbol	Function
sodium	Na^+	Osmotic pressure, nerve impulse transmission
chloride	Cl^-	Osmotic pressure, aids digestion
potassium	K^+	Osmotic pressure, acid–base balance, nerve impulse transmission
calcium	Ca^{2+}	Bone growth and development, blood coagulation, enzyme activity, neuromuscular function
magnesium	Mg^{2+}	Enzyme action in synthesis of ATP, muscle contraction, protein synthesis
phosphate	HPO_4^{2-}, $H_2PO_4^-$	Acid–base balance
bicarbonate	HCO_3^-	Acid–base balance
sulfate	SO_4^{2-}	Acid–base balance
carbonic acid	H_2CO_3	Acid–base balance

neuromuscular function, cardiac **arrhythmias** are often seen in patients with potassium imbalances. A potassium imbalance is of special concern in surgical patients because of increased risk of cardiac arrhythmias or arrest when a general anesthetic is administered. Many elderly patients may be taking diuretics (see Chapter 7) and can easily become hypokalemic, so a potassium level must be determined on all surgical patients taking diuretics. Elective surgery may be postponed until potassium levels have been restored to a safe range.

Sodium (Na^+) controls distribution of water in the body and maintains fluid and electrolyte balance. Sodium is vital to neuromuscular function.

Intravenous Fluids

Appropriate fluid and electrolyte management is an integral component of surgical patient care. Nearly every surgical patient will receive intravenous fluids. Parenteral fluid therapy has three objectives: to maintain daily fluid requirements, to restore previous losses, and to replace current losses. To accomplish these objectives, several fluids are available and are used for specific purposes.

COMMON IV FLUIDS ADMINISTERED IN SURGERY

Sodium chloride, also called normal saline, in a .9% solution (**isotonic**), is the most common IV fluid used in surgery. Sodium chloride is packaged in 1000-, 500-, 250-, and 100-mL bags for IV administration. Sodium chloride is used when chloride loss is greater than or equal to sodium loss, for treatment of **metabolic acidosis** in the presence of fluid loss, to replenish lost sodium, and for mixing with packed red blood cells.

Dextrose is used in patients who require an easily metabolized source of calories. Dextrose is available in various concentrations in water and in normal saline. Dextrose in water is used to hydrate the surgical patient, spare body protein, and enhance liver function. Because the trauma and stress of surgery cause some water and sodium retention, intraoperative intravenous therapy often involves administration of limited amounts of dextrose 5% in water (D5W). Dextrose in water is also prepared in 2.5%, 10%, 20%, and 50% solution.

Dextrose 5% in normal saline (D5NS) is packaged in bags of 1000, 500, 250, and 150 mL. This fluid is used for temporary treatment of circulatory insufficiency and shock due to hypovolemia, in the absence of a plasma extender, and for early treatment with plasma for loss of fluid due to burns. Dextrose 10% in normal saline (D10NS) is supplied in 1000- and 500-mL bags and is used to replenish nutrients and electrolytes.

Lactated Ringer's (LR), or Hartmann's, solution is a physiologic salt solution used to replenish the patient's electrolytes and rehydrate the patient to stimulate renal activity. Lactated Ringer's solution, which is used to replace fluid lost from burns or severe diarrhea, closely resembles the composition of extracellular fluid.

Plasma-lyte and Isolyte E are electrolyte balanced solutions compatible with the pH of blood. They are used to treat the massive loss of water and electrolytes seen in uncontrolled vomiting or diarrhea. The composition of these solutions is similar to the plasma portion of blood. See Table 14–3 for a summary of common intravenous fluids.

INTRAVENOUS EQUIPMENT AND SUPPLIES

An intravenous line is established in nearly all surgical patients prior to surgery. A flexible catheter (Fig.14–5) is inserted via a needle into a vein, usually in the patient's hand or forearm. The needle is removed, leaving the catheter in place. A long tubing is connected to a container of intravenous solution and is inserted into the hub of the catheter and taped securely in place. Fluids and most of the medications needed during surgery are administered through the intravenous line.

Table 14–3 **Common Intravenous Fluids**

Name	Concentration	Abbreviation
Sodium chloride (normal saline)	.9%	NS
Dextrose	5% in water	D5W
	5% in normal saline	D5NS
Lactated Ringer's		LR

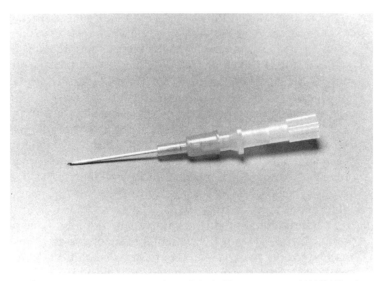

Figure 14–5   Intravenous catheter (Jelco). (Photo courtesy of J&J/Critikon)

Summary

Fluid and electrolyte balance and blood replacement are key components of intraoperative patient management. The surgical technologist must understand the basics of fluid and blood replacement therapy in order to function effectively in the operating room. While surgical technologists do not administer these items, they often assist in many ways. The surgical technologist may obtain products for infusion, set up intravenous lines, prepare blood transfusion supplies and equipment, or operate the cell-saver. Blood replacement therapy is commonplace in surgery and the surgical technologist must understand both the fundamental principles and application of those principles in order to provide competent assistance to the anesthesia provider. Intravenous fluids are given for specific purposes and the surgical technologist should be familiar with various types and uses of IV fluids common to the operating room as well as supplies needed to administer these fluids.

REVIEW

1. What are the basic functions of blood?

2. What is the average circulating blood volume in an adult?

3. What type of surgical patient may need blood replacement?

4. What are the formed elements of blood? What is the main purpose of each?

5. What is hemoglobin? Hematocrit?

6. What is the normal range of hemoglobin in an adult male? An adult female?

7. What is the normal range of hematocrit?

8. How does antigen/antibody reaction pertain to blood types?

9. What are three critical electrolytes? What is the impact of imbalance of each on the surgical patient?

10. What common IV fluids are used in surgery? What is the purpose of each?

11. What supplies are needed to start an intravenous line?

CHAPTER **15**

Anesthesia Complications

OBJECTIVES

Upon completion of this chapter you should be able to:

1 Identify potential complications associated with anesthesia.
2 Match complications with drugs used in treatment of each.
3 Match drugs used in emergency situations with purposes.
4 Discuss the role of the surgical technologist during a cardiac emergency in surgery.
5 List clinical signs of malignant hyperthermia.
6 Outline basic course of treatment for malignant hyperthermia.
7 Discuss the role of the surgical technologist in an MH crisis.
8 Define terminology related to anesthesia complications.

KEY TERMS

Anaphylaxis An unusual or exaggerated allergic reaction of an organism to foreign protein or other substances.

Asystole Cardiac standstill or arrest; absence of heartbeat.

Bolus A concentrated amount of medication administered rapidly intravenously.

Bradycardia Slow heart beat, less than 60 beats per minute.

Bronchospasm Involuntary contraction of the smooth muscle of the bronchi, causing impaired breathing.

Capnography Measurement of inspired and expired carbon dioxide concentrations.

Cyanosis A bluish discoloration of the skin and mucous membranes due to inadequate oxygen in the blood (desaturation).

Desaturation Reduction of oxygen saturation in the blood.

Diaphoresis Perspiration, especially profuse perspiration.

Dyspnea Labored or difficult breathing.

Fulminant Occurring suddenly, with great intensity.

Hemoglobinemia Presence of free hemoglobin in the blood plasma.

Hemoglobinuria Presence of free hemoglobin in the urine.

Hypermetabolic Increased metabolism.

Pyrexia A fever, or febrile condition.

Sympathomimetic Adrenergic; producing effects resembling those impulses transmitted by the sympathetic nervous system.

Tachycardia Abnormally rapid heart rate, greater than 100 beats per minute.

Tachypnea Very rapid respirations, greater than 30 per minute.

Urticaria A vascular reaction of the skin marked by transient appearance of slightly elevated patches (wheals) that are redder or paler than the surrounding skin and often attended by severe itching.

The administration of any anesthetic is a complex process, and can be associated with several complications. These potential complications, which vary from mild to life-threatening, are unusual, but merit careful study by the surgical technologist. Several anesthesia complications require treatment with emergency drugs, which will be discussed in this chapter. Two of the most pertinent to the surgical technologist—cardiac arrest and malignant hyperthermia—will be discussed at length. The complications discussed are not necessarily exclusive to anesthesia; rather, they may be attributed to the condition of the surgical patient or the surgical procedure itself.

Anesthesia Complications

Anaphylaxis

Anaphylactic shock (**anaphylaxis**) may result from a severe allergic reaction to medications, anesthetics, or blood administered in surgery. Anaphylactic shock occurs rapidly and is potentially lethal. Early signs include hives and **urticaria** (wheals), followed by respiratory obstruction, **dyspnea** (labored breathing), circulatory collapse, and severe **bronchospasm** (impaired breathing due to contraction of the bronchi). If signs of anaphylaxis appear, any medications being administered should be discontinued and a dose of diphenhydramine (Benadryl) given intravenously. Diphenhydramine (Benadryl, Allergan 50) is an antihistamine; it is used to treat allergic reactions or as an adjunct in treatment of anaphylaxis. Normal dosage is .2–.5 mg/kg IV. If this treatment is effective, surgery may continue, but without the use of the suspected agent. If conservative treatment is not effective, the allergic reaction may quickly progress to anaphylaxis and possible cardiac arrest. In such case, a "code blue" is called and emergency resuscitation measures are taken. Oxygen is administered, epinephrine is given, and sometimes sodium bicarbonate and aminophylline. Aminophylline is used to treat bronchoconstriction seen in anaphylaxis and acute asthma attacks. The exact method of action is not clear, but it relaxes the bronchial smooth muscle, allowing better ventilation. Aminophylline is administered IV 5–6 mg/kg over a period of 20–30 minutes. Aminophylline is gradually being replaced by proventil (Albuterol).

Agents that cause the most frequent allergic reactions include penicillin, codeine, contrast media, morphine, meperidine, thiopental, and tubocurarine.

Transfusion Reaction

Blood and blood products are at times transfused during a surgical procedure. Any adverse reaction to the administration of blood or blood products in surgery is a condition treated and managed by the anesthesia provider. Numerous safety precautions are taken during all phases of blood replacement to ensure that the patient receives only compatible blood. Rarely, however, the patient may experience a transfusion reaction due to administration of incompatible blood. A transfusion reaction may be characterized by fever, urticaria, hypotension, **hemoglobinemia** (hemoglobin in plasma), **hemoglobinuria** (hemoglobin in urine), shock, and disseminated intravascular coagulopathy (DIC). Transfusion reactions are usually treated with antipyretics and antihistamines, such as diphenhydramine, in addition to discontinuation of the blood products.

Respiratory Obstruction

Respiratory obstruction may be caused by a number of factors including swelling due to trauma or inflammation, bronchospasm, laryngospasm, or asthma. Aminophylline is used to treat acute asthma attacks, prevent bronchoconstriction in asthmatics, and reverse bronchospasm when seen in patients with chronic obstructive pulmonary disease (COPD).

Laryngospasm

Laryngospasm may occur shortly after extubation as a reaction to removal of the endotracheal tube. Laryngospasm is seen more frequently in children and infants, and is characterized by a high-pitched crowing sound on inspiration. Positive airway pressure is administered in an effort to break the spasm. If the spasm does not respond to pressure, and pulse oximetry shows oxygen **desaturation,** a dose of succinylcholine (Anectine, Quelicin) will be given IV or IM to relax the muscles of the larynx. (For further discussion of succinylcholine, see Chapter 13.) Reintubation may be necessary in order to achieve adequate oxygenation.

Vomiting and Aspiration

Several anesthetic agents in use today cause nausea. If the patient is sufficiently nauseated, vomiting may occur. Vomiting is not as dangerous in an awake patient because the cough reflex allows the patient to clear his or her own airway of vomitus. In a patient under general anesthesia, however, vomiting may be a life-threatening situation; inability to clear the airway may result in aspiration of gastric contents into the lungs. Due to its acidic nature, the gastric contents can severely damage delicate lung tissue. This condition is called *aspiration pneumonia.* Depending on the extent of damage, the patient may be admitted for observation and treated with antibiotics if febrile. Antacids and antiemetic drugs may be administered preoperatively to reduce the risk of vomiting and aspiration. For elective surgical procedures, routine orders include nothing by mouth (NPO) for 4–8 hours prior to scheduled surgery to reduce the volume of gastric contents.

Fluid and Electrolyte Imbalances

Due to the nature of drugs administered to produce anesthesia, some electrolyte imbalances may occur. Recall that fluid electrolytes most crucial to homeostasis include sodium, calcium, and potassium (see Chapter 14). Electrolyte imbalances are usually managed by administration of intravenous fluids specifically formulated to treat the problem. For instance, a patient who is dehydrated will receive intravenous sodium chloride (NaCl) or Lactated Ringer's solution. A patient who is hypokalemic may be given IV potassium preoperatively to prevent cardiac arrhythmias.

Emergency Situations

The surgical technologist should be able to respond appropriately to any patient emergency. In order to function in a competent manner, the surgical technologist must have a thorough knowledge of the drugs frequently used in emergency situations. The pertinent pharmacology of two emergency situations seen in surgery will be discussed at length.

Cardiac Arrest

Cardiac arrest may occur at any time before, during, or after an anesthetic. A cardiac arrest may be attributed to several causes. For example, some anesthetic agents can cause cardiac irritability or arrhythmias; in other cases, the patient may have an existing condition, such as cardiac disease or a low serum potassium, that might precipitate a cardiac arrest.

If a cardiac arrest does occur in the operating room, the surgical technologist should know exactly what to do in order to assist in providing competent patient care. Cardiac or respiratory arrest in surgery is usually called a "code blue" or "code 99." A crash cart containing emergency medications and a cardiac defibrillator (Fig. 15–1) should be immediately available and brought into the operating room. The surgical technologist may perform several roles during a cardiac arrest. In the circulating role, the surgical technologist may notify appropriate personnel of the situation, bring in or call for the crash cart, assist the anesthesia provider, and/or perform cardiac compressions as needed. In the scrub role, the surgical technologist may need to remain sterile to cover or close the wound if necessary, prepare the internal defibrillator paddles for use, or prepare to open the chest cavity for open-heart massage. If a second surgical technologist is scrubbed, he or she may be asked to break scrub to obtain the crash cart. He or she may also be designated as the official record keeper, recording all medications given, dosages, and times of events on a special form provided on the crash cart. It is vital that the surgical technologist be familiar with medications given during a cardiac emergency, their usual dosages, and their purposes. The following is a brief synopsis of drugs frequently used in treatment of a cardiac arrest (Table 15–1).

Atropine sulfate is a cholinergic antagonist used to block the effects of the vagus nerve on the sino-atrial (SA) node of the heart. Atropine or a similar drug,

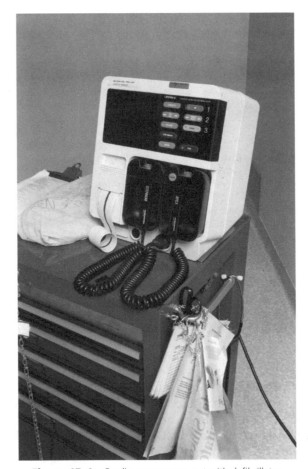

Figure 15–1 Cardiac emergency cart with defibrillator.

glycopyrrolate (Robinul), may be given IV in doses of .4–1.0 mg (adult) preoperatively (Chapter 12) to prevent **bradycardia** arising from a vagal response to such stimuli as stretching of the peritoneum or placing traction on eye muscles. If **asystole** occurs as a response to such actions, a code blue is called and cardiac resuscitation is initiated. Additional amounts of atropine may be injected during the resuscitation process.

Epinephrine hydrochloride (Adrenalin) is a hormone (Chapter 9) that acts as a cardiac stimulant. Epinephrine is also a bronchodilator, and may be used to treat allergic reactions. During a cardiac arrest, epinephrine may be injected directly into heart muscle (intracardiac) in an effort to restore both force and rate of myocardial contractions. Intravenous dosage is usually a .5–1.0 mg **bolus**, which may be repeated every 5 minutes as needed. Epinephrine is also used in non-emergency situations to prolong the duration of local anesthetics (Chapter 13).

Table 15–1 Summary of Cardiac Emergency Drugs

Generic Name	Trade Name	Purpose
Aminophylline	Aminophylline	Bronchospasm, asthma
Atropine sulfate	Atropine	Bradycardia, asystole
Calcium chloride		Increase force of myocardial contractions
Dantrolene sodium	Dantrium	Malignant hyperthermia
Digoxin	Lanoxin	Atrial tachycardia, atrial fibrillation, slow heart rate, strengthen myocardial contractions
Diphenhydramine	Benadryl	Anaphylaxis
Epinephrine	Adrenalin	Cardiac stimulant; anaphylaxis
Isoproterenol	Isuprel	Arrhythmias, resuscitation, stabilize heart rate, strengthen contractions, bradyarrhythmias
Lidocaine	Xylocaine	Premature ventricular contractions (PVCs), ventricular tachycardia, ventricular arrhythmias
Norepinephrine	Levophed	Restore blood pressure
Procainamide	Procan SR, Pronestyl	Arrhythmias in MH, atrial fibrillation, paroxysmal atrial tachycardia, treatment of lidocaine-resistant ventricular arrhythmias
Sodium bicarbonate		Metabolic acidosis
Verapamil	Calan, Isoptin	Calcium channel blocker; treat tachyarrhythmias, angina; antihypertensive

Sodium bicarbonate is used to treat metabolic acidosis, which is frequently seen in cardiac arrest. Sodium bicarbonate neutralizes excess hydrogen ion concentration in the blood, thus raising blood pH. In cardiac arrest, sodium bicarbonate is given IV 1 mEq/kg and repeated 0.5 mEq/kg every 10 minutes during the arrest.

Miscellaneous Cardiac Drugs

Calcium chloride is an electrolyte replacement given to increase the force of myocardial contractions. Dosage is 10 mg/kg IV in a 2%–10% solution.

Digoxin (Lanoxin) is a cardiac glycoside used to increase the force of myocardial contractions. It is also used to treat congestive heart failure (CHF), atrial fibrillation and flutter, and paroxysmal atrial tachycardia (PAT). Digoxin is administered IV, .5–1.0 mg in divided doses.

Isoproterenol hydrochloride (Isuprel) is a **sympathomimetic** agent administered to increase the rate and force of myocardial contractions. It is also used to treat bradyarrhythmias and serves as a bronchodilator.

Lidocaine hydrochloride (Xylocaine) is a local anesthetic given intravenously to treat ventricular arrhythmias such as premature ventricular contractions (PVCs), especially those associated with acute myocardial infarction or cardiac surgery. Lidocaine in a 1% or 2% solution is administered slowly IV in doses of 1 mg/kg. This may be repeated .5 mg/kg every 2–5 minutes as needed.

Norepinephrine bitartrate (Levophed) is a potent peripheral vasoconstrictor used to raise blood pressure, subsequently increasing coronary artery blood flow. Levophed is administered IV .04–.4 mcg/kg/min.

Verapamil hydrochloride (Isoptin) is a calcium channel blocker used to treat tachyarrhythmias and angina. It is also used as an antihypertensive agent.

☞ Many different drugs may be used during a cardiac emergency, and only the most common are introduced here. It is strongly suggested that the surgical technology student review an actual crash cart at a local clinical facility to further study the medications used to treat cardiac arrest.

Malignant Hyperthermia

Malignant hyperthermia (MH) is a rare anesthesia complication. It is crucial, however, that the surgical technologist understand the signs, treatment and pharmacology involved in such a crisis in order to function as a competent surgical team member.

Malignant hyperthermia is defined as a **fulminant hypermetabolic** crisis triggered by some anesthetic agents. If untreated, mortality is nearly 80%. Agents known to trigger this disease are succinylcholine (Anectine) and all inhalation anesthetics except nitrous oxide.

CLINICAL SIGNS OF MALIGNANT HYPERTHERMIA

Contrary to popular belief, **pyrexia** is NOT an early indicator of malignant hyperthermia (Table 15–2). A rise in patient temperature indicates that a full crisis is in effect. The earliest sign presented will be an increase in end-tidal carbon diox-

Table 15–2 Clinical Signs of Malignant Hyperthermia

Increase in end-tidal CO_2
Tachycardia
Tachypnea
Masseter muscle rigidity (MMR)
Unstable blood pressure
Arrhythmias
Cyanosis
Diaphoresis
Pyrexia

ide. An increase of even 5 mm/Hg could be significant. End-tidal CO_2 can increase for several reasons other than MH; but when other possibilities have been ruled out, the anesthesia provider may begin to alert the operating room staff that potential exists for an MH crisis.

Additional early signs include **tachycardia** and **tachypnea.** These conditions may have other causes as well; but in combination with the signs described here, tachycardia and tachypnea are classic symptoms of MH. Both tachycardia and tachypnea are means the body uses to eliminate the excess carbon dioxide that is accumulating due to the hypermetabolic crisis. Tachypnea may even override the ventilator setting.

Muscle rigidity, especially masseter muscle rigidity (MMR), can be an early warning of MH; but there are other, benign causes of MMR. Opinions vary on the correlation here; but if MMR is present, the patient should be closely monitored for MH. In combination with signs described above, MMR is considered a classic sign of MH.

In addition, the patient may exhibit an unstable blood pressure, arrhythmias, **cyanosis**, **diaphoresis**, and a rapid increase in body temperature. Temperatures of more than 42°C have been reported.

Once MH has been triggered, the patient can die in as little as 15 minutes, so prompt diagnosis and treatment are vital.

MALIGNANT HYPERTHERMIA TREATMENT PROTOCOL

Once MH has been identified, the surgical procedure will be stopped if possible and all anesthetic agents will be discontinued. The patient will be hyperventilated with 100% oxygen, to help eliminate the excess CO_2 that accumulates in the blood. Ventilator tubing will be changed to prevent exposure to residual inhalation agents. Dantrolene sodium (Dantrium), a skeletal muscle relaxant developed specifically to treat MH, will be administered IV. Initial dosage is 2.5 mg/kg. Dantrolene is packaged, freeze-dried, in vials of 20 mg with 3000 mg of mannitol, and must be reconstituted with 60 mL of sterile water. In an adult patient weighing 80 kg (176 lb), 200 mg of dantrolene (10 vials) will be required to begin treatment. Dosages may reach 10 mg/kg, so in this case 800 mg (40 vials) of dantrolene may need to be reconstituted. If appropriate, the scrubbed surgical technologist may break scrub to help reconstitute the dantrolene. Once sterile water has been injected into the vial, the mixture must be shaken vigorously until the solution becomes clear yellow, indicating complete reconstitution. Dantrolene is administered until symptoms disappear. Malignant hyperthermia may also be seen in children, so the number of vials reconstituted will be adjusted accordingly. Sodium bicarbonate will be given IV to treat the metabolic acidosis resulting from high concentrations of lactate in the blood. Blood gasses will be monitored frequently. The patient must be rapidly cooled to prevent brain damage. Ice packs will be applied to groin, neck, and axilla in an effort to lower the temperature. Iced lavage of stomach, rectum, and/or bladder may be performed to cool the patient's core temperature. Diuretics such as mannitol (Osmitrol) or furosemide (Lasix) will be given IV to keep the kidneys functioning properly. Muscle cells are destroyed during an MH crisis, and the myoglobin that is released in this process tends to accumulate in the kidneys, obstructing flow. Procainamide or lidocaine will be given IV to treat arrhythmias secondary to electrolyte imbalances. Procainamide (Procan SR, Pronestyl) is an antiarrhythmic agent used to control arrhythmias seen in malignant hyperthermia; it is also used to treat atrial fibrillation, lidocaine-resistant ventricular arrhythmias, and paroxysmal atrial tachycardia (PAT). Lidocaine is also used as an antiarrhythmic. Glucose and insulin will be administered to treat hyperkalemia, frequently seen because potassium (K^+) is released as muscle cells are destroyed. All of these treatment steps will be taken virtually simultaneously, and are arranged to help remember key points. All patient vital functions will be monitored closely to determine response to treatment. **Capnography** is crucial, as are arterial lines, frequent blood gas assessment, and accurate temperature measurement. A Foley catheter should be in place to measure urine output. Basic treatment steps for a malignant hyperthermia crisis are summarized in Table 15–3. For additional information, call or write:

Malignant Hyperthermia Association of the United States
PO Box 1069
Sherburne, NY 13460
Phone (607)-674-7901

A hotline staffed by volunteer physicians has been established to assist with information to treat an MH crisis:

1-(800)-MH HYPER
[1-(800)-644-9737]

Treatment can be considered successful when vital signs and blood gases return to within normal limits. Elective surgery will be discontinued. Life-threatening surgery will be resumed, but with different anesthetic agents and a different anesthesia machine to prevent residual inhalation agent from triggering a second crisis. Upon cancellation or completion of the surgical procedure, the patient will be transported to the intensive care unit (ICU) or PACU accom-

Table 15–3 Malignant Hyperthermia
Treatment Steps

Hyperventilate—with 100% oxygen
Dantrolene—administer 2.5–10 mg/kg IV
Sodium bicarbonate—IV to treat metabolic acidosis
Temperature management—ice packs and lavage
Diuretics—Mannitol or furosemide IV

panied with the replenished MH cart, as another episode could yet occur. Always consult and follow individual institution policies covering an MH crisis. The surgical technologist should become familiar with all institutional policies covering any emergency situation, including MH. In addition, the surgical technologist should be familiar with signs, treatment, and pharmacology of malignant hyperthermia.

Summary

Any patient receiving an anesthetic is at risk for potential complications. Some complications treated pharmacologically include anaphylactic shock, fluid and electrolyte imbalances, respiratory obstruction, and vomiting with potential for aspiration. While not common occurrences in surgery, these situations merit careful study and continuing education. As an allied health professional, the surgical technologist must attain and maintain the proficiency required to function effectively in these emergency situations. Cardiac arrest and malignant hyperthermia are of particular importance to the surgical technologist. Some drugs used to treat anesthesia emergencies include aminophylline, atropine, calcium chloride, Dantrium, Lanoxin, Benadryl, epinephrine, Isuprel, lidocaine, Levophed, procainamide, sodium bicarbonate, and verapamil.

Malignant hyperthermia is defined as a fulminant hypermetabolic crisis triggered by some anesthetic agents. Signs of an MH crisis include tachycardia, tachypnea, masseter muscle rigidity, unstable blood pressure, arrhythmias, cyanosis, diaphoresis, and pyrexia. Basic treatment steps for malignant hyperthermia are hyperventilation with 100% oxygen, intravenous injection of dantrolene and sodium bicarbonate, temperature management, and administration of diuretics.

REVIEW

1. What are some anesthesia complications treated pharmacologically?

2. What are the drugs used to treat those complications?

3. Why is vomiting so dangerous to the surgical patient?

4. Can you name some drugs used to treat cardiac arrest? What is the purpose of each?

5. What are the signs of malignant hyperthermia?

6. What are the basic treatment steps for MH?

7. How would the circulating surgical technologist function during a cardiac emergency or a malignant hyperthermia crisis? As first scrub? As second scrub?

APPENDIX

Antineoplastic Chemotherapy Agents

KEY TERMS

Antineoplastic Agents that inhibit malignant or cancerous cells.

Benign Noncancerous or nonmalignant; favorable recovery.

Cancer Common term given to neoplastic diseases that involve turning normal body cells into malignant ones.

Cytotoxic Agents destructive to all dividing cells.

Malignant Cancerous; tending to become progressively worse and to result in death. Having the properties of invasiveness and metastasis.

Metastasis The transfer of disease from one organ or part to another not directly connected with it.

Neoplasm Tumor; any new and abnormal growth of cells. May be benign or malignant.

Cancer

The term **cancer** is a common one in the surgical setting. Nearly one-third of all Americans will be affected by some type of cancer during their lives. It may be found in any age group, but is more often seen in older people. As the years of human life expectancy continue to increase, there is more evidence of cancer.

Before cancer can start, a disruption (possibly in the cell's genetic material) must occur which transforms normal cells into **malignant** ones. Normal body cells divide and multiply in order to replace dying ones. When this rate of cell division is disrupted and not controlled, an abnormal growth of cells is formed. This abnormal growth is called a tumor, or **neoplasm.** Neoplasms may be **benign,** which means they resemble normal tissue, grow slowly, are highly organized cells, and do not normally spread into surrounding tissue. These tumors may be surgically removed if they disrupt normal body functions or cause pain. Neoplasms may also be malignant, or cancerous. These cells are unorganized and immature, multiply rapidly, and invade surrounding tissues. They can travel through the circulatory or lymphatic systems and spread to other areas of the body where they form another tumor called a **metastasis.** Many times, surgery is performed to diagnose and/or remove cancerous tumors. However, surgery may not be the only treatment required in order to cure the patient of the disease.

Chemotherapy Agents

Pharmaceutical agents play an important role in the treatment of cancer outside of the surgical setting. **Antineoplastic** agents can be used as systemic treatment in the primary or main tumor, and in its metastases. This is often in addition to surgical treatment. These agents are **cytotoxic** and thus affect normal cells as well as malignant ones. They are often given intravenously in high doses on an established schedule. This allows normal cells to recover in between chemotherapy drug doses. Antineoplastic agents are used for remission or palliative effects. Remission is the abatement (stopping) of symptoms and possible cure of the disease. Palliative means the relief of symptoms without cure. Antineoplastic agents are classified according to their mechanism of actions: alkylating agents, antimetabolites, natural products such as plant alkaloids, antineoplastic antibiotics, and hormones. Steroids are also used along with antineoplastics to help prevent nausea and vomiting—a common side effect of chemotherapy. Other side effects include diarrhea, bone marrow depression, rashes, alopecia (hair loss), and scaling of the skin. Antineoplastic agents are contraindicated in pregnancy and in patients with renal or hepatic disorders. Types of cancers associated with chemotherapy in conjunction with surgical treatment include breast and prostate cancers. Common antineoplastic agents are fluorouracil (5FU), methotrexate (Mexate), cyclophosphamide (Cytoxan), bleomycin (Blenoxane), and paclitaxel (Taxol). It should be noted that continued advancements are being made in this field. Often combination chemotherapy is standard in tumor treatment (antineoplastic agents used in combinations and regimens).

☞ Other terminology for cancer includes carcinoma and the initials CA.

Index

Note: Page numbers in *italics* refer to illustrations; page numbers followed by t refer to tables.